Strategies to Protect the Health of Deployed U.S. Forces

Force Protection and Decontamination

Michael A. Wartell, Michael T. Kleinman,
Beverly M. Huey, and Laura M. Duffy, *Editors*

Strategies to Protect the Health of Deployed U.S. Forces:
Physical Protection and Decontamination

Division of Military Science and Technology
Commission on Engineering and Technical Systems

National Research Council

NATIONAL ACADEMY PRESS
Washington, D.C.

NOTICE: The project that is the subject of this report was approved by the Governing Board of the National Research Council, whose members are drawn from the councils of the National Academy of Sciences, the National Academy of Engineering, and the Institute of Medicine. The authors responsible for the report were chosen for their special competencies and with regard for appropriate balance.

This is a report of work supported by Contract DASW01-97-C-0078 between the National Academy of Sciences and the Department of Defense. Any opinions, findings, conclusions, or recommendations expressed in this publication are those of the author(s) and do not necessarily reflect the view of the organizations or agencies that provided support for the project.

International Standard Book Number 0-309-06793-6

Limited copies are available from:

Board on Army Science and Technology
National Research Council,
2101 Constitution Avenue, N.W.
Washington, D.C. 20418
(202) 334-3118

Additional copies are available from:

National Academy Press
2101 Constitution Ave., N.W.
Box 285
Washington, D.C. 20055
800-624-6242/202-334-3313
(in the Washington metropolitan area)

Copyright 1999 by the National Academy of Sciences. All rights reserved.

Printed in the United States of America.

THE NATIONAL ACADEMIES

National Academy of Sciences
National Academy of Engineering
Institute of Medicine
National Research Council

The **National Academy of Sciences** is a private, nonprofit, self-perpetuating society of distinguished scholars engaged in scientific and engineering research, dedicated to the furtherance of science and technology and to their use for the general welfare. Upon the authority of the charter granted to it by the Congress in 1863, the Academy has a mandate that requires it to advise the federal government on scientific and technical matters. Dr. Bruce M. Alberts is president of the National Academy of Sciences.

The **National Academy of Engineering** was established in 1964, under the charter of the National Academy of Sciences, as a parallel organization of outstanding engineers. It is autonomous in its administration and in the selection of its members, sharing with the National Academy of Sciences the responsibility for advising the federal government. The National Academy of Engineering also sponsors engineering programs aimed at meeting national needs, encourages education and research, and recognizes the superior achievements of engineers. Dr. William A. Wulf is president of the National Academy of Engineering.

The **Institute of Medicine** was established in 1970 by the National Academy of Sciences to secure the services of eminent members of appropriate professions in the examination of policy matters pertaining to the health of the public. The Institute acts under the responsibility given to the National Academy of Sciences by its congressional charter to be an adviser to the federal government and, upon its own initiative, to identify issues of medical care, research, and education. Dr. Kenneth I. Shine is president of the Institute of Medicine.

The **National Research Council** was organized by the National Academy of Sciences in 1916 to associate the broad community of science and technology with the Academy's purposes of furthering knowledge and advising the federal government. Functioning in accordance with general policies determined by the Academy, the Council has become the principal operating agency of both the National Academy of Sciences and the National Academy of Engineering in providing services to the government, the public, and the scientific and engineering communities. The Council is administered jointly by both Academies and the Institute of Medicine. Dr. Bruce M. Alberts and Dr. William A. Wulf are chairman and vice chairman, respectively, of the National Research Council.

STRATEGIES TO PROTECT THE HEALTH OF DEPLOYED U.S. FORCES: FORCE PROTECTION AND DECONTAMINATION

Principal Investigators

MICHAEL T. KLEINMAN, University of California, Irvine
MICHAEL A. WARTELL, Indiana University-Purdue University Fort Wayne

Advisory Panel

WYETT H. COLCLASURE II, Environmental Technologies Group, Inc., Baltimore, Maryland
STEPHEN HILL, Global Analytics, Inc., Orange, Virginia
SIDNEY A. KATZ, Rutgers University, Camden, New Jersey
FRANK K. KO, Drexel University, Philadelphia, Pennsylvania
HOWARD IRA MAIBACH, University of California, San Francisco
NAJMEDIN MESHKATI, University of Southern California, Los Angeles

Board on Army Science and Technology Liaison

JOSEPH J. VERVIER, ENSCO, Inc., Melbourne, Florida

Staff

BRUCE A. BRAUN, Director, Division of Military Science and Technology
BEVERLY M. HUEY, Study Director
LAURA M. DUFFY, Research Associate
PAMELA A. LEWIS, Senior Project Assistant
ANDRE MORROW, Senior Project Assistant

Department of Defense Liaisons

MICHAEL KILPATRICK, Office of the Special Assistant for Gulf War Illnesses, Falls Church, Virginia
FRANCIS L. O'DONNELL, Office of the Special Assistant for Gulf War Illnesses, Falls Church, Virginia

BOARD ON ARMY SCIENCE AND TECHNOLOGY

WILLIAM H. FORSTER, chair, Northrop Grumman Corporation, Baltimore, Maryland
THOMAS L. MCNAUGHER, vice chair, RAND Corporation, Washington, D.C.
ELIOT A. COHEN, School of Advanced International Studies, Johns Hopkins University, Washington, D.C.
RICHARD A. CONWAY, Union Carbide Corporation (retired), Charleston, West Virginia
GILBERT F. DECKER, Walt Disney Imagineering, Glendale, California
PATRICK F. FLYNN, Cummins Engine Company, Inc. Columbus, Indiana
EDWARD J. HAUG, NADS and Simulation Center, The University of Iowa, Iowa City, Iowa
ROBERT J. HEASTON, Guidance and Control Information Analysis Center (retired), Naperville, Illinois
ELVIN R. HEIBERG, III, Heiberg Associates, Inc., Mason Neck, Virginia
GERALD J. IAFRATE, University of Notre Dame, Notre Dame, Indiana
DONALD R. KEITH, Cypress International, Alexandria, Virginia
KATHRYN V. LOGAN, Georgia Institute of Technology, Atlanta, Georgia
JOHN E. MILLER, Oracle Corporation, Reston, Virginia
JOHN H. MOXLEY, Korn/Ferry International, Los Angeles, California
STEWART D. PERSONICK, Drexel University, Philadelphia, Pennsylvania
MILLARD F. ROSE, NASA Marshall Space Flight Center, Huntsville, Alabama
GEORGE T. SINGLEY, III, Hicks and Associates, Inc., McLean, Virginia
CLARENCE G. THORNTON, Army Research Laboratories (retired), Colts Neck, New Jersey
JOHN D. VENABLES, Venables and Associates, Towson, Maryland
JOSEPH J. VERVIER, ENSCO, Inc., Melbourne, Florida
ALLEN C. WARD, Ward Synthesis, Inc., Ann Arbor, Michigan

Staff

BRUCE A. BRAUN. Director
MICHAEL A. CLARKE, Associate Director
MARGO L. FRANCESCO, Staff Associate
CHRIS JONES, Financial Associate
DEANNA SPARGER, Senior Project Assistant

COMMISSION ON ENGINEERING AND TECHNICAL SYSTEMS

W. DALE COMPTON *chair*, Purdue University, West Lafayette, Indiana
ELEANOR BAUM, Cooper Union for the Advancement of Science and Art, New York, New York
RUTH M. DAVIS, Pymatuning Group, Inc., Alexandria, Virginia
HENRY J. HATCH, (U.S. Army retired), Fluor Daniel Hanford, Inc., Richland, Washington
STUART L. KNOOP, Oudens and Knoop, Architects, PC, Chevy Chase, Maryland
NANCY G. LEVESON, Massachusetts Institute of Technology, Cambridge
CORA B. MARRETT, University of Massachusetts, Amherst
ROBERT M. NEREM, Georgia Institute of Technology, Atlanta
LAWRENCE T. PAPAY, Bechtel Technology and Consulting, San Francisco, California
BRADFORD W. PARKINSON, Stanford University, Stanford, California
JERRY SCHUBEL, New England Aquarium, Boston, Massachusetts
BARRY M. TROST, Stanford University, Stanford, California
JAMES C. WILLIAMS, GE Aircraft Engines, Cincinnati, Ohio
RONALD W. YATES, (U.S. Air Force retired), Monument, Colorado

Staff

DOUGLAS BAUER, Executive Director
DENNIS CHAMOT, Deputy Executive Director
CAROL R. ARENBERG, Technical Editor

Preface

Chemical and biological (CB) warfare has been the subject of numerous studies supported by a wide spectrum of sponsoring groups, ranging from the military to private sector foundations. Given how much has already been said on the subject, one might conclude that little remains on which to comment. However, the subject is complex and controversial enough that with each new hostile military encounter, with each potential new threat, with each report of a possible terrorist action using CB agents, our defensive preparedness comes under new scrutiny.

The military experience in the Gulf War, while overwhelmingly positive by almost any measure, raised some concerns. One obvious uncertainty was that there might be a causal relationship between the presence of CB agents in theater and the symptoms reported by returning military personnel, later named the "Gulf War Syndrome." Studies focused initially on whether personnel might have been exposed to low-level doses of chemical agents, and if this exposure could have resulted in the reported symptoms. More recent studies have been expanded to cover the whole range of CB defense, from medical issues to materiel development to doctrine and training.

Responding to the need for an evaluation of the military's ability to prosecute missions in CB environments, the Department of Defense Office of the Special Assistant for Gulf War Illnesses, through the National Academies, sponsored a study of strategies to protect the health of deployed U.S. forces, focused on CB defense. The first part of this three-year study was divided into four parallel studies (1) to develop an analytical framework for assessing the risks to deployed forces; (2) to review and evaluate technologies and methods for detection and tracking exposures to those risks; (3) to review and evaluate physical protection and decontamination; and (4) to review and evaluate medical protection, health consequences and treatment, and medical record keeping. Now, at the end of the second year of the study, each group is providing a report to DoD and the public on its findings and recommendations in these areas. These four documents will be used as a basis for a new National Academies consensus committee that will prepare a synthesis report for DoD in the third year of the project. The consensus committee will consider, not only the topics covered in the four two-year studies, but also overarching issues relevant to its broader charge.

This report responds to the third of the first four studies, physical protection and decontamination. The task, which is more fully described in the first chapter, includes (1) an assessment of DoD's approaches and technologies for physical protection—both individual and collective—against CB warfare agents and decontamination of personnel and equipment, and (2) an assessment of DoD's current policies, doctrine, and training. The issues of space, budget, and staffing allocations for these programs, although extremely important, are beyond the scope of this report. Unlike most National Academies studies, two principal investigators conducted this study, with the assistance and guidance of an advisory panel. The expertise of this advisory panel covered various topics addressed by the study.

During the data-gathering phase, we received extensive briefings, visited various facilities, consulted with numerous experts, solicited commissioned papers on specialized topics, attended many related national conferences and symposia, and reviewed other material provided by DoD and from the open literature. We also held one workshop to gather additional information on focussed topics. We are indebted to the organizations and individuals that gave freely of their time and talents to this project. A special note of thanks to the individuals, listed by name, appears in Appendix F of this report. Given the countless individuals who shared their expertise with us, there is no doubt the list is incomplete; and we apologize for the oversights.

In responding to our Statement of Task, we attempted to cover each aspect of the requested information, adding introductory and historical information. No single study, however, can do justice to the entire breadth of topics included in our study charge. Therefore, we decided to focus on issues on which we believed we could provide especially helpful advice to the military.

During the course of the study, we were struck by several aspects of the CB defense community: (1) their dedication to their professions, in general, and to CB protection, in particular; (2) the extent to which decades-old threat information continues to influence current requirements and considerations; (3) the willingness of policy makers to accept "worst case" assessments against which to develop programs, as opposed to developing more valid benchmarks based on more up-to-date information; (4) the continuing need for basic science information on the chemical, physical, and toxicological properties of CB agents to facilitate the development of modeling and simulations; (5) the need for more and better uses of modeling and simulations; and (6) the contrast between the high quality doctrine and training approaches available and inconsistent CB training across services and across units.

We wish to emphasize that the CB defense community is competent, caring, and dedicated. Although we suggest areas for improvement in this report, we retain a strongly positive overall impression of the work of the CB community.

The individuals who reviewed the draft report were especially important to the construction of the final report. They provided thoughtful and constructive comments that significantly enhanced the quality of the final report. Finally, we gratefully acknowledge the work and support of Beverly Huey, the National Academies study director for this project. Her dedication, intelligence, and flexibility were invaluable and are deeply appreciated. We also thank Laura Duffy, the research associate, for her efforts in acquiring and organizing data that were central to our analyses.

Michael T. Kleinman
Michael A. Wartell
Principal Investigators

Strategies to Protect the Health of Deployed U.S. Forces:
Physical Protection and Decontamination

Acknowledgments

We are appreciative of the cooperation we received from the many individuals and organizations who provided valuable information and guidance to us in the course of our work. First, we extend our sincere thanks to the members of the advisory panel who provided assistance and guidance during the information gathering process, gave thought-provoking presentations in their respective areas of expertise, participated in briefings from various organizations, and provided thoughtful comments on the initial drafts of this report. We are also indebted to those individuals who prepared commissioned papers for our use: William Hinds, who wrote a paper on respiratory protection; Sidney Katz on air contaminant removal; Frank Ko on textiles and garments for chemical and biological protection; Howard I. Maibach and Hongbo Zhai on barrier creams, percutaneous absorption, and skin decontamination techniques; and Maher Todios on decontamination.

We are grateful for the guidance and support from others at the National Academies, including Joseph Cassells and Suzanne Woolsey, who assisted in the coordination of the four separate study efforts as they were simultaneously being conducted; Bruce Braun, who assisted in scoping the study, nurtured it throughout its execution and provided ongoing oversight; and Douglas Bauer and Dennis Chamot, who adeptly dealt with stumbling blocks when they occurred in the process and provided thoughtful insights throughout the course of the study. We also appreciate the work of Pamela Lewis who provided administrative assistance in preparing this document for review and publication, and Carol Arenberg, who edited this document, enhancing its clarity. Finally, we are indebted to numerous other NRC staff for their individual contributions: Mike Clarke, associate division director; Margo Francesco, staff associate; Delphine Glaze, Jacqueline Campbell-Johnson, and Andre Morrow, senior project assistants; and Alvera Wilson, financial associate.

Without the extensive contributions and thought-provoking comments so freely given by so many individuals throughout the course of this study, we could not have completed the task set before us. We would like to acknowledge those individuals who provided briefings, arranged site visits to their organizations, gave presentations at the workshop, supplied invaluable information and reports critical to our charge, answered our searching questions very honestly, and assisted us in contacting other sources who could provide additional information and documentation not easily accessible. There is no doubt the list is incomplete, and we apologize for any oversights (see Appendix F).

This report has also been reviewed by individuals chosen for their diverse perspectives and technical expertise, in accordance with procedures approved by the National Research Council's Report Review Committee. The purpose of this independent review is to provide candid and critical comments that will assist the authors and the National Research Council in making the published report as sound as possible and to ensure that the report meets institutional standards for objectivity, evidence, and responsiveness to the study charge. The content of the review comments and draft manuscript remain confidential to protect the integrity of the deliberative process. We wish to thank the following individuals for their participation in the review of this report:

Robert E. Boyle, Department of the Army (retired)
Gerald T. Dinneen, Honeywell, Inc. (retired)
Stephen W. Drew, Merck & Co., Inc.
Valerie J. Gawron, Veridian Engineering
Trevor J. Little, North Carolina State University
John Nelson, NBC Defense Systems (retired)
Donald F. Petersen, Department of Defense Health Effects Programs (retired)
Ellen Raber, Lawrence Livermore National Laboratory
William G. Reifenrath, Reifenrath Consulting & Research
Bruce O. Stuart, Schering-Plough Research Institute

While all of the advisors and reviewers listed above have provided many constructive comments and suggestions, responsibility for the final content of this report rests solely with the authoring principal investigators and the National Research Council.

Contents

EXECUTIVE SUMMARY	1
1 INTRODUCTION	16
Background of the Study, 18	
Charge to the National Academies, 19	
Scope of the Study, 19	
Limitations, 20	
Approach of the Study, 21	
Overview of the Report, 21	
2 THREAT AND RISK ASSESSMENT	23
Historical Perspective of the Chemical/Biological Battle Space, 23	
U.S. Response, 26	
Relationships among Policy; Doctrine; Research, Development and Acquisition; and Threat, 29	
Contamination Avoidance, 31	
Individual Protection, 31	
Collective Protection, 32	
Decontamination, 32	
Medical Systems, 32	
Characteristics of Current and Future Chemical and Biological Agents, 32	
Effects and Tactical Utility of Chemical Agents, 32	
Effects and Tactical Utility of Biological Agents, 34	

Proliferation of Chemical and Biological Agents, 36
Production, Weaponization, and Dispersion, 38
Threatened Use of Chemical and Biological Weapons, 39
Assessment of Chemical and Biological Warfare Risks, 39
   Hazards: Routes and Levels of Exposure, 40
   Threat Assessment, 52
Risk Minimization/Protection of Personnel, 53
Findings and Recommendation, 56

3 PHILOSOPHY, DOCTRINE, AND TRAINING FOR CHEMICAL AND BIOLOGICAL WARFARE   58
Philosophy, 58
Chemical/Biological Warfare Doctrine, 60
   Past Doctrine: "Fight Dirty," 60
   Current Doctrine: Contamination Avoidance, 61
Chemical/Biological Warfare Training, 61
Understanding the Risk, 63
Findings and Recommendations, 66

4 PHYSICAL PROTECTION   67
Individual Protection, 67
   Risks and Challenges, 67
   Current Doctrine and Training, 68
   Textiles and Garments, 73
   Barrier Creams, 89
   Impacts on Effectiveness, 89
   Patient Protective Equipment, 93
   Summary, 94
Collective Protection, 94
   Risks, Challenges, and Requirements, 94
   Filters, 95
   Filter Systems, 95
   Protective Structures and Systems, 97
Advanced Filters and Adsorbents, 99
   Filters, 100
   Absorbers, 101
   Service-Life Indicators, 102
   Regeneration, 103
   Catalytic Oxidation, 103
Findings and Recommendations, 104

CONTENTS   xv

5 DECONTAMINATION   108
   Decontamination of Skin, 110
      Risks and Challenges, 110
      Technologies, 111
   Decontamination of Equipment, Facilities, and Large Areas, 113
      Risks and Challenges, 113
      Technologies, 113
      Reactions and Mechanisms, 117
   Current Doctrine and Training, 132
Findings and Recommendations, 136

6 TESTING AND EVALUATION   138
   Toxicological Testing, 138
      Evaluation of Percutaneous Penetration, 139
      Evaluation of Barrier Creams, 143
   Test Equipment, 143
   Predictive Models and Simulations, 149
   Exercises and Systems Evaluations, 149
   Findings and Recommendations, 150

7 ASSESSMENT OF MILITARY CAPABILITIES TO
   PROVIDE EMERGENCY RESPONSE   151
   Findings and Recommendations, 153

8 SUMMARY AND GENERAL RECOMMENDATIONS   155
   Threat, 156
   Policy, Doctrine, and Training, 157
   Chemical/Biological Protective Equipment, 157
      Threat-Based Requirements and the Development of
         Equipment, 157
      Physical Protection, 159
      Decontamination, 160
      Testing, 161
      Program Objective Memorandum for Funding
         Research, 162
      Summary, 163

REFERENCES   164

APPENDICES

A Funding Levels   181
B Textiles and Garments for Chemical and Biological Protection   182

C Evaluations of Barrier Creams	217
D Evaluating Skin Decontamination Techniques	221
E Percutaneous Absorption	224
F Contributors to This Study	230
G Biographical Sketches of Principal Investigators and Members of the Advisory Panel	236

Tables, Figures, and Box

TABLES

2-1 Integrated CINC Priorities, 29
2-2 Nuclear, Biological, Chemical (NBC) Nonmedical Defense Program Priorities, 30
2-3 Categorization of Chemical Agents, 33
2-4 Categorization of Biological Agents, 35
2-5 Inhalation/Respiratory Agents, 42
2-6 Dermal Absorption Agents, 46
2-7 Dermal Necrotic Agents, 48
2-8 Inhalation/Respiratory Agents, 48
2-9 Ingestion Agents, 50
2-10 Agents Absorbed via Mucous Membranes or the Skin, 50
2-11 Arthropod Vectors, 52
2-12 Time to Achieve MOPP 4, 54
2-13 Levels of Mission-Oriented Protective Posture (MOPP), 55

3-1 Service Requirements for JSLIST, 63

4-1 Approximate Toxicity of Chemical Agents, 69
4-2 Time to Achieve MOPP 4, 71
4-3 Requirements for Chemical Protective Textiles, 74
4-4 Evolution of Performance Requirements for Protective Textiles, 75
4-5 Summary of Required Improvements in Fibrous Material Properties, 76

| 4-6 | Requirements for the C2 Air-Purification Device, 100 |

5-1	Differences between the Decontamination of Fixed Sites and Mobile Forces, 109
5-2	Decontamination Coatings, 114
5-3	Characteristics of Oxidizing Decontaminants, 120
5-4	Advantages and Disadvantages of Enzymatic Decontamination, 125
5-5	Military Air Guidelines for Chemical Warfare Agents, 135

| 6-1 | Efficacy of Barrier Creams, 144 |

FIGURES

| 2-1 | Management structure of the DoD Chemical and Biological Defense Program, 28 |

| 3-1 | Summary of appropriations for the Chemical and Biological Defense Program, 59 |

| 4-1 | Construction of a selectively permeable barrier, 77 |
| 4-2 | Components of a typical current barrier system, 78 |

5-1	Secondary products formed by hydrolysis of sulfur mustard, 118
5-2	Catalytic acceleration of soman by iodobenzoate, 118
5-3	Oxidation of VX in acidic solution, 122
5-4	Molecular approaches to enhancing the solubility of chemical agents in liquid media, 123
5-5	Decontamination of paper treated with 25 mg VX per 25 cm^2, 126
5-6	^{31}P NMR study of the decontamination of O-ethyl-S-ethyl phenyl phosphonothioate, 127
5-7	Foam decontamination of *Bacillus subtilis* spores after one hour of treatment, 128
5-8	(a) High-energy accelerator fitted on a truck. (b) Schematic drawing of large-area decontamination with ionizing radiation, 132

BOX

| 2-1 | Persistence of Biological Agents, 36 |

Abbreviations and Acronyms

ABBREVIATIONS

2D	two dimensional
3D	three dimensional
cfm	cubic foot per minute
CG	phosgene
Cl	chlorine
CK	cyanogen chloride
Ct	concentration × time
CX	phosgene oxime
D_{10}	the dose level required to reduce the sample population by a factor of 10
DS2	decontaminating solution number 2
DS2P	propylene glycol monomethyl ether
ECt_{50}	the Ct dose that causes a defined effect (e.g., edema or death) in 50 percent of a given population
GA	tabun
GB	sarin
GD	soman
g/den	gram per denier

H	Levinstein mustard
H2S	hydrogen sulfide
HD	distilled mustard
HL	mustard-lewisite mixture
HN	nitrogen mustard
ICt_{50}	the Ct dose that incapacitates 50 percent of a given population
ID_{50}	the dose that incapacitates 50 percent of a given population
L	Lewisite
lpm	liters per minute
MeV	million electron volts
m^2/g	square meter per gram
$mg \times min/m^3$	milligram times minute per cubed meter
mm	millimeter
nm	nanometers
NO_x	nitrogen oxides
ppb	parts per billion
$\Omega\text{-}kg/m^2$	ohm kilogram per square meter

ACRONYMS

AERP	aircrew eye/respiratory protection
ALERT	attack and launch early reporting to theater
ASTM	American Society for Testing and Materials
AUIB	aircrew uniform integrated battlefield
BDO	battle dress overgarment
BDU	battle dress uniform
BWC	Biological and Toxic Weapons Convention
CB	chemical and/or biological
CBIRF	Chemical Biological Incident Response Force
CINC	commander-in-chief
CONUS	continental United States
CPE	collective protection equipment
CPU	chemical protective undergarment

CWC	Chemical Weapons Convention
DARPA	Defense Advanced Research Projects Agency
DATSD (CP/CBD)	Deputy Assistant to the Secretary of Defense for Counter-proliferation and Chemical/Biological Defense
DEPMEDS	deployable medical system
DoD	U.S. Department of Defense
DMMP	dimethyl methylphosphate
DPD	dermatopharmacodynamic
DPK	dermatopharmacokinetic
ERDEC	Edgewood Research, Development, and Engineering Center (now known as the Chemical-Biological Center of Excellence of the Soldier and Biological Chemical Command)
FF	fit factor
FM	field manual
FOC	functional operational capability
FR	flame resistance
FY	fiscal year
ICBPG	improved chemical and biological protective glove
IOM	Institute of Medicine
JCS	Joint Chiefs of Staff
JPO-BD	Joint Program Office for Biological Defense
JSAPE	joint service aircrew protective ensemble
JSAM	joint service aircrew mask
JSGPM	joint service general purpose mask
JSIG	Joint Service Integration Group
JSLIST	joint service lightweight integrated suit technology
JSMG	Joint Service Materiel Group
LCBPG	lightweight chemical/biological protective garment
LRC	lesser regional conflicts
LSC	liquid scintillation counting
MAG	military air guideline
MCBAT	Medical Chemical-Biological Advisory Team
MIST	Man-in-Simulant Test (program)

MLRS	multiple launch rocket system
MNS	mission needs statement
MOPP	mission-oriented protective posture
MRC	major regional conflicts
MULO	multipurpose rain/snow/CB overboot
MURI	multidisciplinary university research initiative
NATO	North Atlantic Treaty Organization
NBC	nuclear, biological, chemical
NMR	nuclear magnetic resonance
OOTW	operations other than war
OPAA	organophosphorous acid anhydrolase
OPH	organophosphorous hydrolase
P3I	preplanned product improvement (program)
PF	protection factor
POM	program objective memorandum
PPE	personal protective equipment
PVC	polyvinyl chloride
R&D	research and development
RDA	research, development and acquisition
RDIC	resuscitation device individual chemical
RDT&E	research, development, test and evaluation
RSDL	reactive skin decontaminant lotion
SAW	surface acoustic wave
SBCCOM	Soldier and Biological Chemical Command
SCALP	suit, contamination avoidance, liquid protection
SLS	sodium lauryl sulfate
SMART-CB	special medical augmentation response team–chemical/biological
SMART-PM	special medical augmentation response team–preventative medicine
SRT	Specialty Response Team
STEPO	self-contained toxic environment protective outfit
TAP	toxicological agent protective
TEMPER	tent, expandable modular personnel
TG	technical guide
VHP	vapor of hydrogen peroxide
VPU	vapor protective undergarment

Strategies to Protect the Health of Deployed U.S. Forces

Executive Summary

Since Operation Desert Shield/Desert Storm, Gulf War veterans have expressed concerns that medical symptoms they have experienced could have been caused by exposures to hazardous materials or other deployment-related factors associated with their service during the war. Potential exposure to a broad range of chemical and/or biological (CB) and other harmful agents was not unique to Gulf operations but have been a component of all military operations in this century. Nevertheless, the Gulf War deployment focused national attention on the potential, but uncertain, relationship between the presence of CB agents in theater and health symptoms reported by military personnel. Particular attention has been given to the potential long-term health effects of low-level exposures to CB agents.

Since the Gulf War, U.S. forces have been deployed to Haiti, Somalia, Bosnia, Southwest Asia, and, most recently, Kosovo, where they were (and are) at risk of exposure to toxic CB threats. The U.S. Department of Defense (DoD) anticipates that deployments will continue in the foreseeable future, ranging from peacekeeping missions to full-scale conflicts. Therefore, the health and preparedness of U.S. military forces, including their ability to detect and protect themselves against CB attack, are central elements of overall U.S. military strength. Current doctrine requires that the military be prepared to engage in two simultaneous major regional conflicts while conducting peacekeeping operations and other assignments around the globe. The diversity of potential missions, as well as of potential threats, has contributed to the complexity of developing an effective strategy.

BACKGROUND

In the spring of 1996, Deputy Secretary of Defense John White met with the leadership of the National Academies to discuss the DoD's continuing efforts to improve protection of military personnel from adverse health effects during deployments in hostile environments. Although many lessons learned from previous assessments of Operation Desert Shield/Desert Storm have been reported, prospective analyses are still needed: (1) to identify gaps and shortcomings in policy, doctrine, training, and equipment; and (2) to improve the management of battlefield health risks in future deployments.

DoD determined that independent, external, unbiased evaluations focused on four areas would be most useful: (1) health risks during deployments in hostile environments; (2) technologies and methods for detecting and tracking exposures to harmful agents; (3) physical protection and decontamination; and (4) medical protection, health consequences and treatment, and medical record keeping. This report, which addresses the issues of physical protection and decontamination, is one of four initial reports that will be submitted in response to that request.

CHARGE

This study, conducted by two principal investigators with the support of an advisory panel and National Academies staff from the Commission on Engineering and Technical Systems, assessed DoD approaches and technologies that are, or may be, used for physical protection—both individual and collective—against CB agents and for decontamination. This assessment includes an evaluation of the efficacy and implementation of current policies, doctrine, and training as they relate to protection against and decontamination of CB agents during troop deployments and recommends modifications in strategies to improve protection against deleterious health effects in future deployments. This report includes reviews and evaluations of the following topics:

- current protective equipment and protective measures, as well as those in development
- current and proposed methods for decontaminating personnel and equipment after exposure to CB agents
- current policies, doctrine, and training for protecting against and decontaminating personnel and equipment in future deployments
- the effects of using current protective equipment and procedures on unit effectiveness and other human performance factors
- current and projected military capabilities to provide emergency response to terrorist CB incidents

THREAT AND RISK ASSESSMENT

Chemical and Biological Battle Space

Chemical agents were first used extensively as military weapons during World War I. CB weapons programs continued to flourish during the 1950s and 1960s, led by scientists in the United States and the Soviet Union, and to a lesser extent, in other countries including Great Britain. New nerve agents were developed during those years, including the family of V agents, which are not only lethal in smaller ingested doses but can also be absorbed directly through the skin. Natural toxins and biological pathogens were also investigated as biological warfare agents.

In the post-1950s era, improving the means of dissemination of lethal agents became a major research objective. Airborne spray tanks, specialized artillery shells, CB-capable missile warheads, and an assortment of other weapons were developed. The United States discontinued its offensive biological and chemical military research programs in 1969 and 1989, respectively, but continued to expand its defensive programs. However, CB technologies have continued to proliferate in other countries, and with advances in bioengineering and molecular biological capabilities, even small nations or groups now have the potential to develop novel biological agents. This asymmetrical threat prompted the United States to extend its CB defense programs, which have increased substantially since Desert Shield/Desert Storm.

The estimated CB threat from Soviet forces during the Cold War was based on the perceptions that a broad range of chemical and biological weapons had been fielded, that the Soviet Union had the capability of deploying and supporting those weapons on the battlefield, and that the Soviets were pursuing an extensive research program. U.S. tactics, training, and requirements were based on this perceived threat. Today, many countries possess CB capabilities although intelligence assessments indicate that most of them have limited quantities of agents and limited delivery systems.

Response to Chemical/Biological Threats

The CB threat to U.S. forces can be defined as the perceived capability of an opposing force to expose U.S. forces to CB agents. The most obvious way to minimize the risk of CB exposure is to avoid contact with these materials. Therefore, the military has developed a doctrinal principle for protecting deployed forces based on avoiding exposure (i.e., contamination avoidance). Avoiding contact depends on the capability and availability of detection equipment; however, because of current lag times in detection capability, a responsive strategy (the so-called "detect to treat" strategy), rather than a preventive strategy, has been necessary.

The U.S. intelligence community provides data, analyses, and advice concerning the development of CB capabilities by threat nations. Based on this information, commanders and the Joint Service Integration Group (JSIG) evaluate how CB agents could be used against U.S. troops and develop policy, doctrine, training, and requirements for equipment to counter the perceived threat. As the threat changes, U.S. approaches to countering the threat should also change.

As a result of the proliferation of CB capabilities, recent reductions in U.S. forces, continuing budget constraints, and attempts to minimize duplications of effort among the services, operations have become more integrated and cooperative (i.e., joint service operations). To encourage the integration of CB research and development (R&D) at all levels, in 1994 Congress enacted Public Law 103-160, the National Defense Authorization Act for Fiscal Year 1994 (Title XVII), establishing a new structure for the CB defense program.

Finding. Joint structure and joint service processes were developed to maximize the efficient use of funds and reduce duplications of effort.

Finding. The object of the joint prioritization of system needs (and, therefore, research, development, and acquisition [RDA] needs) is to ensure that fielded systems meet joint service needs. This requires that commander-in-chief (CINC) priorities and nuclear, biological, chemical (NBC) community priorities be coordinated.

Finding. The prioritization and selection of RDA projects are often based on compromises or political trade-offs unrelated to CINC prioritization, technical capabilities, or bona fide needs and are focused on service-specific rather than joint service needs.

Recommendation. The Department of Defense should reevaluate and possibly revise its prioritization process for the development of equipment. The reevaluation should include reassessment of the use of threat information.

Challenge

The chemical agent challenge established for protective equipment ($10g/m^2$ for liquids; 5,000–10,000 $mg\text{-}min/m^3$ for vapors) has not been changed in four decades. Although analyses using relatively sophisticated computer models have shown that under certain conditions,

10 g/m² levels may be present in localized areas of a battlefield, the average concentration may be considerably lower. These same models predict that the areas where levels would be higher than 10 g/m² would be the same areas where the shrapnel and projected shell materials would be more likely to cause injuries or deaths than CB agents. Nevertheless, because challenge levels determine the requirements for protection, the goals of the entire CB R&D program are based on the 10 g/m² level for liquid agents and 5,000–10,000 mg-min/m³ for vaporous agents.

Finding. The battlefield areas with the highest contamination levels will also have the highest levels of ballistic fragmentation lethalities. Therefore, CB protective measures will be ineffective in these areas regardless of the liquid or vapor challenge levels. The threat from CB weapons relative to other battlefield threats is unknown.

Finding. System development is sometimes based on outdated and possibly inaccurate evaluations of threats and challenges.

Recommendation. The Department of Defense should reevaluate the liquid and vapor challenge levels based on the most current threat information and use the results in the materiel requirements process and, subsequently, in the development of training programs and doctrine.

Finding. Little or no new funding is being provided for basic research on new technologies for physical protection or decontamination.

Recommendation. The Department of Defense should reprogram funds to alleviate the shortfall in basic research on new technologies for physical protection and decontamination.

PHILOSOPHY, DOCTRINE, AND TRAINING

The CB defense program involves (1) contamination avoidance (reconnaissance, detection, and warning); (2) force protection (individual and collective protection and medical support); and (3) decontamination. Before systems for detecting contaminated areas were available, military planners developed a doctrine (best described as the "fight dirty" doctrine) that was based on conducting operations in contaminated areas. Implementing the doctrine involved providing a combination of individual protective equipment and extensive training on fighting in contaminated environments. As technology has advanced, especially detection technologies, and as new detection equipment has been fielded, the doctrine has shifted to "contamination avoidance." Stated simply, this doctrine provides that U.S. forces will engage an enemy while avoiding casualties from contamination by CB agents.

Once the doctrine of contamination avoidance (with concomitant detection and protective equipment) was adopted, training was naturally modified to carry out the new doctrine. A critical requirement for deterring the use of CB agents (and for successful operations if deterrence fails) is that forces be fully trained to respond to the full spectrum of CB threats. Operational requirements must balance the risk factors from all sources and determine trade-offs between protecting the individual and maintaining the combat effectiveness of the force.

Finding. The current doctrine is based on the concept of contamination avoidance, although U.S. CB detection systems do not, as a rule, provide sufficient advance warning to prevent exposures.

Finding. Unit commanders receive little training related to assessing CB risks to their units, especially in determining when, whether, and how much protective gear is necessary.

Recommendation. The Department of Defense should develop commander training protocols and/or simulations to assist unit leaders in making appropriate chemical and biological risk-based decisions.

INDIVIDUAL PROTECTION

The military conceptual approach to individual protection, called mission-oriented protective posture (MOPP), is an ensemble comprised of protective garments, boots, masks, and gloves. MOPP levels proceed (i.e., adding parts of the ensemble) from the MOPP-ready level to the MOPP 4 level, increasing the level of protection in response to the hazard. Because design requirements for personal protective equipment (PPE) include the ability to withstand the established threat and risk levels, PPE has severely limited individual (and unit) performance. Problems include difficulties in speech and communications, impairment in hearing, reduced vision, thermal stress, occasional adverse reactions to materials, and overall reductions in operational effectiveness.

Some improvements in PPE have been made, however. For example, the joint service lightweight integrated suit technology (JSLIST) affords better CB protection, reduces the physiological heat burden, and interferes less with weapons systems than previous technologies. The JSLIST preplanned product improvement (P3I) should provide even better protection. Because the human respiratory system is extremely vulnerable to the highly toxic and rapidly acting agents to which deployed forces may be exposed, respiratory protection is a major factor in contamination avoidance. Respirators of various types have been developed and used both in military and civilian operations. The newest mask—the joint service general purpose mask (JSGPM)—allows better peripheral vision, is reasonably comfortable to wear, and has a somewhat flexible design to meet service-specific requirements.

The hands have traditionally been protected by impermeable gloves; however, recent research has also focused on multilaminate technologies and barrier creams designed to prevent or reduce the penetration and absorption of hazardous materials by the skin, thus preventing skin lesions and/or other toxic effects. Effective barrier creams might also be used to protect skin adjacent to areas where the garments are known to provide less than optimal protection (e.g., under seams, around closures).

Finding. Current challenges used to evaluate protective equipment do not reflect changes in threat levels.

Recommendation. The Department of Defense should reevaluate its requirements for materiel development to protect against liquid and vapor threats and revise design requirements, if appropriate.

Finding. PPE modules (e.g., masks, garments, gloves) were designed as independent items and then "retrofitted" to create an ensemble. They were also developed without adequate attention to various human factors issues, such as the integration of PPE with weapon systems.

Finding. The most serious risk from most CB agents appears to be from inhalation. Current doctrine allows for Mask-Only protection, but the mask seal could be broken while advancing from Mask-Only to MOPP 4 status.

Recommendation. A total systems analysis, including human factors engineering evaluations, should be part of the development process of the personal protective equipment system to ensure that the equipment can be used with weapon systems and other military equipment. These evaluations should include:

- the performance of individuals and units on different tasks in various realistic scenarios
- the interface of the mask and garments and potential leakage during an "advance" from Mask-Only to MOPP 4 status

Finding. Although researchers have good data from human factors testing that identified serious performance (cognitive and physical) limitations as a result of wearing PPE, they have been unable to adequately relate these deficiencies to performance on the battlefield.

Recommendation. The Department of Defense should place greater emphasis on testing in macroenvironments and controlled field tests rather than relying mostly on systems evaluations for personal protective equipment.

Finding. Although the seal of the mask is much improved over previous mask models, seal leakage continues to be a critical problem. The leakage can be attributed to (1) problems with the interface between the seal and the face, and (2) improper fit.

Recommendation. Additional research is needed on mask seals and mask fit. The research program should focus on seals, fit, and sealants (adhesives). The duration/severity of leaks, if any, during transitions in protective posture from one MOPP level to another should also be investigated. These data would be useful for future studies on long-term health effects of low-level exposures. In addition, training to fit masks properly should be conducted for all deployed forces equipped with mission-oriented protective posture equipment.

Finding. Although mask fit testing has been shown to improve protection factors 100-fold, the Air Force and Army have only recently begun deploying mask fit testing equipment and providing appropriate training protocols and supportive doctrine.

Recommendation. Doctrine, training, and equipment for mask fit testing should be incorporated into current joint service operations. The Department of Defense should deploy the M41 Mask Fit Test kit more widely.

Finding. Leakage around closures in personal protective equipment remains a problem.

Recommendation. The Department of Defense should continue to invest in research on new technologies to eliminate problems associated with leakage around closures. This research could include the development of a one-piece garment, the use of barrier creams on skin adjacent to closure areas, and other technologies still in the early stages of development.

EXECUTIVE SUMMARY 9

Finding. Current gloves reduce tactile sensitivity and impair dexterity.

Recommendation. The Department of Defense should evaluate using a combination of barrier creams and lightweight gloves for protection in a chemical and/or biological environment. Multilaminate gloves should also be further explored.

Finding. An impermeable garment system is believed to provide the most comprehensive protection against CB agents. But impermeable barriers cause serious heat stress because they trap bodily moisture vapor inside the system. Permeable systems, which breathe and allow moisture vapor to escape, cannot fully protect against aerosol and liquid agents.

An incremental improvement could be achieved by using a semipermeable barrier backed with a sorptive layer. This system would allow the moisture vapor from the body to escape and air to penetrate to aid in cooling. The multilayer system would have some disadvantages, however. It would be bulky and heavy. The sorptive layer is an interstitial space where biological agents could continue to grow because human sweat provides nutrients for biological agents, which could prolong the period of active hazards. Countermeasures should be investigated to mitigate these problems.

Recommendation. The Department of Defense should investigate a selectively permeable barrier system that would be multifunctional, consisting of new carbon-free barrier materials, a reactive system, and residual-protection indicators.

The carbon-free barrier materials could consist of: (1) smart gel coatings that would allow moisture/vapor transport and would swell up and close the interstices when in contact with liquid; (2) selectively permeable membranes that would allow moisture/vapor transport even in the presence of agents; (3) electrically polarizable materials whose permeability and repellence could be electronically controlled.

The reactive material could be smart, carbon-free clothing with gated membranes capable of self-decontamination. A reactive coating could also be applied to the skin in the form of a detoxifying agent (e.g., agent reactive dendrimers, enzymes, or catalysts capable of self-regeneration).

A residual-protection indicator would eliminate the premature disposal of serviceable garments and might also be able to identify the type of contamination. Conductive polymers could be used with fiber-optic sensors to construct the device.

COLLECTIVE PROTECTION

Collective protective structures (e.g., shelters and positive pressure vehicles) provide relatively unencumbered safe environments where activities such as eating, recovery, command and control, and medical treatment can take place. Collective protective equipment is based on filtering and overpressurization technologies. Advanced filters and adsorbents are critical components in these systems. Improvements in protection will depend on the availability of advanced filtration and adsorbent capabilities.

Finding. The Department of Defense does not have enough collective protection units to meet the needs of deployed forces.

Recommendation. The Department of Defense should assess the needs of deployed forces for collective protection units in light of changing threats and the development of new personal protective equipment and provide adequate supplies of such equipment to deployed forces.

DECONTAMINATION

Decontamination is the process of neutralizing or removing chemical or biological agents from people, equipment, and the environment. For military purposes, decontamination must restore the combat effectiveness of equipment and personnel as rapidly as possible. Most current decontamination systems are labor intensive and resource intensive, require excessive amounts of water, are corrosive and/or toxic, and are not considered environmentally safe. Current R&D is focused on the development of decontamination systems to overcome these limitations and effectively decontaminate a broad spectrum of CB agents from all surfaces and materials. Because of the vastly different characteristics of personnel, personal equipment, interior equipment, exterior equipment, and large outdoor areas, situation-specific decontamination systems must be developed.

DoD has developed doctrine and training for decontamination but has not established levels of acceptable risk. Therefore, detection capabilities are not designed to verify acceptable decontamination levels.

Finding. Just as only a few benchmarks for the removal of MOPP gear have been established (because detection technology is inadequate), few benchmarks of decontamination levels have been established. Therefore, it is difficult to know when it is safe to return equipment to operational status and impossible to "certify" that previously contaminated equipment

EXECUTIVE SUMMARY 11

can be transported to a new location, especially a location in the United States.

Recommendation. The Department of Defense should initiate a joint service, interagency, and international cooperative effort to establish decontamination standards. Standards should be based on the best science available and may require the development of new models for setting benchmarks, especially for highly toxic or pathogenic agents.

If residual decontamination levels are based on ultraconservative toxicity and morbidity estimates, returning contaminated equipment becomes impractical. Benchmarks for decontamination should be based on highly accurate, reliable, up-to-date toxicity data.

Finding. Although significant progress is being made with limited resources in exploring decontamination technologies that may be effective, no organized, integrated research program has been developed to meet the new challenges and objectives that have been posed (i.e., environmentally acceptable decontamination). Various agencies are actively pursuing many projects, but they are not well coordinated and do not have clear priorities for fixed-site programs, casualty management, and sensitive equipment programs.

Recommendation. The Department of Defense (DoD) should coordinate and prioritize the chemical/biological research and development (R&D) defense program, focusing on the protection of deployed forces and the development of environmentally acceptable decontamination methods. DoD should also establish the relative R&D priority of decontamination in the chemical/biological defense program.

Finding. Recent developments in catalytic/oxidative decontamination (enzymes, gels, foams, and nanoparticles) appear promising for decontaminating a wide range of CB agents.

Recommendation. Research on enzyme systems for battlefield decontamination (especially for small forces) should be given high priority because they could be used to decontaminate both personnel and equipment and would not require large volumes of water or complicated equipment.

Recommendation. The Department of Defense should continue to develop other catalytic/oxidative systems for larger scale decontamination. If possible, these systems should be less corrosive and more environmentally acceptable than current methods.

Finding. Low-power plasma technology has been shown to be effective for decontaminating sensitive equipment and has the potential of incorporating contaminant-sensing capabilities.

Recommendation. The Department of Defense should continue to develop plasma technology and other radiation methods for decontaminating equipment.

TESTING AND EVALUATION

Testing and evaluation of equipment, methodologies, and the toxicological effects of chemical agents are critical for the development of appropriate defensive strategies. Adherence to the principles of the nonproliferation agreements entered into by the United States prohibits most tests using live agents, as well as studies with human volunteers (except with surrogate agents). Most human and animal tests are, therefore, conducted using simulants, although it is not entirely clear that these simulants are adequate surrogates.

The most comprehensive test program, the Man-in-Simulant Test (MIST) Program, which tests complete and partial protective ensembles under controlled conditions, is a valuable program, although it has many shortcomings. Simulants are commonly used for testing protective and decontaminating equipment to determine the effectiveness of the protective equipment. However, the simulants have not been systematically validated to determine how closely their behavior mimics the behavior of actual agents. Therefore, the United States may not have the ability to determine whether or not a specific piece of equipment actually meets its performance requirements.

Finding. Testing of dermatological threat agents has not been consistent. The available quantitative data are not sufficiently precise to make an accurate evaluation of potential percutaneous threats from agents other than blister agents or irritants.

Recommendation. Tests of dermatological threat agents should be conducted to establish the level of protection necessary to provide adequate margins of safety and to establish quantitative criteria for evaluating the performance of protective equipment, such as gloves, undergarments, and overgarments.

Finding. Mask testing under the MIST program was unreliable because the passive dosimeters did not function satisfactorily in the mask environment.

Recommendation. Active samplers or improved passive samplers for mask testing using simulants should be developed and made available for tests of the joint service lightweight integrated suit technology (JSLIST) ensemble.

ASSESSMENT OF MILITARY CAPABILITIES TO PROVIDE EMERGENCY RESPONSE

Various initiatives have been implemented and numerous studies undertaken to determine the role and assess the capability of the U.S. military in providing emergency response capabilities in coordination with other federal, state, and local agencies. Examples of military programs to support emergency response include the DoD Chemical Biological Rapid Response Team, the U.S. Army Medical Research Institute of Chemical Defense Chemical Casualty Site Team, the Marine Corps Chemical Biological Incident Response Force, and the National Guard Rapid Assessment and Initial Detection Program.

Finding. Because numerous agencies will respond to a domestic CB incident, close coordination will be necessary for the response to be efficient and effective. Unless civilians (e.g., first responders, employees of relevant state and local agencies, etc.) who respond to domestic CB incidents are equipped with protective and decontamination equipment that is compatible with the equipment used by the military, coordination will be difficult if not impossible.

Recommendation. The Department of Defense, in collaboration with civilian agencies, should provide compatible equipment and training to civilians (e.g., first responders, employees of relevant state and local agencies, etc.) who respond to domestic chemical and/or biological incidents to ensure that their activities can be coordinated with the activities of military units. Doctrine and guidance must be developed on an interagency basis.

Finding. Doctrine and training are not well developed for mission-critical civilians working at military installations that might become targets of chemical and/or biological attacks.

Recommendation. Coordinated doctrine, training, and guidance on individual protective equipment, collective protective equipment, and decontamination should be established on a joint service, interagency, and coalition basis for civilians working at military installations.

SUMMARY AND GENERAL RECOMMENDATIONS

The health of military personnel who served in the Gulf War, and of personnel who will serve in future deployments, is a matter of great concern to veterans, the public, Congress, and DoD. Based on the many lessons that have been learned from the Gulf War and subsequent deployments, as well as on information from other sources, a great deal can be done to minimize potential adverse health effects from exposure to CB agents and to increase protection levels against them.

Recommendation. Threat projections and risk perceptions should be reevaluated in terms of realistic or credible battlefield risks. The requirements for protective equipment should then be adjusted to respond to those threats and challenges.

Characterizing a "low-level" contaminated environment is still an open question. Answering this question has become an urgent priority since post-Gulf War medically unexplained symptoms have become a serious issue. Information on the effects of extended exposures to low levels of CB agents is incomplete, but recent studies have suggested that low-level exposures may have some long-term consequences.

Recommendation. Research on the toxicology of low-level, long-term exposures to chemical and biological agents and other potentially harmful agents (e.g., environmental and occupational contaminants and toxic industrial chemicals) should be continued and expanded.

Unfortunately, modeling and simulation can only partly compensate for the lack of data based on actual experiments. Evidence has shown that modeling and simulation of the performance of CB protective equipment have not been very effective.

Recommendation. The use of simulants, data from animal models, and data on human exposure should be reevaluated as part of the development of a coherent research program to determine the physiological effects of both high-level and low-level long-term exposures to chemical and biological agents. The data should then be used to determine risks and challenges.

Training for CB operations has been very inconsistent, both within and among the services.

Recommendation. Required levels of training (with the appropriate level of funding for training devices and simultants) should be established and monitored for effective unit performance throughout the services. Objective criteria should be established for determining whether current service-specific training requirements are being met.

1

Introduction

The use of chemical and/or biological (CB) agents as weapons dates back many centuries; however, extensive use of these agents as weapons in military conflict began in World War I. Since then, research programs on chemical warfare agents, followed by research on biological agents, have been undertaken by a number of countries, including the United States, Japan, Germany, Italy, and the United Kingdom. Many countries, including the United States, believed that chemical warfare was no more cruel than any other kind of warfare and, thus, should not be banned. During World War II, the United States adopted a "no first use" policy but warned that retaliation against those who did use CB agents would be quick and extensive.

The United States discontinued its offensive biological and chemical military research programs in 1969 and 1989, respectively, but continued to expand its defensive programs. (In fact, the defensive program has been increased substantially since Desert Shield/Desert Storm.) During the Cold War, the perceived CB threat posed by the Soviet Union was based on three factors: (1) the broad range of chemical and biological weapons believed to be possessed by Soviet forces; (2) their ability to deploy and support CB weapons on the battlefield; (3) and the extensive research program apparently being pursued in the Soviet Union. U.S. tactics, training, and requirements were based on responding to this threat.

Since the end of the Cold War, the perceived military threats to the

United States have changed, but the tactics, training, and requirements for CB defense have not changed, although little rationale has been presented for retaining them. Although the threat from the former Soviet Union has significantly lessened, some experts believe that Russia has maintained its arsenal for CB warfare. In addition, more than a dozen other countries (e.g., China, North Korea, India) have been developing technologies and offensive CB capabilities that may pose military threats, but these technologies and capabilities are not as advanced as the technologies and capabilities of the former Soviet Union (Commission to Assess the Organization of the Federal Government to Combat the Proliferation of Weapons of Mass Destruction, 1999).

Because the United States expects to be able to project power globally, the health and preparedness of its military forces, including their ability to detect and protect themselves against CB attack, are central elements of overall U.S. military strength (Payne, 1998). Current doctrine requires that the military be prepared to engage successfully in two simultaneous major regional conflicts while conducting peacekeeping operations and other assignments around the globe. Uncertainty about the future requires that U.S. strategy be adaptable, and the diversity of potential missions, as well as potential threats, have contributed to the complexity of developing a strategy (Secretary of Defense, 1999).

Since Desert Storm, the joint services have mandated that troops receive predeployment and postdeployment health assessments. For the purpose of joint health surveillance, in the December 4, 1998, memorandum the chairman of the Joint Chiefs of Staff (JCS) issued the following official definition of a deployment:

> A troop movement resulting from a JCS/unified command deployment order for 30 continuous days or greater to a land-based location outside the United States that does not have a permanent U.S. military medical treatment facility (i.e., funded by the Defense Health Program). Routine shipboard operations that are not anticipated to involve field operations ashore for over 30 continuous days are exempt from the requirements for pre- and post-deployment health assessments.

Subsequent to Operation Desert Shield/Desert Storm, U.S. forces have been deployed to Haiti, Somalia, Bosnia, Southwest Asia, and, most recently, Kosovo. During these deployments, our forces could have been or may be exposed to CB attacks. This report evaluates our current ability to protect our forces from CB exposures (excluding medical protection, such as vaccines) and assesses improvements in force protection through the development and implementation of doctrine, tactics, techniques, procedures, and training.

BACKGROUND OF THE STUDY

Since Operation Desert Shield/Desert Storm, Gulf War veterans have expressed concerns that their postdeployment medical symptoms could have been caused by hazardous exposures or other deployment-related factors. Potential exposure to a broad range of CB and other harmful agents was not unique to Gulf operations. Hazardous exposures have been a component of all military operations in this century. Nevertheless, the Gulf War deployment focused national attention on the potential, but uncertain, relationship between the presence of CB agents in theater and symptoms reported by military personnel. Particular attention has been given to the potential long-term health effects of low-level exposures to CB agents. As a result, a number of studies have been undertaken addressing the health of veterans and the potential health effects of their service.

At least six different panels (the Defense Science Board Task Force on Persian Gulf War Health Effects; the National Institutes of Health Technology Assessment Workshop; the Institute of Medicine (IOM) Committee on Health Consequences of Service in the Persian Gulf; the Institute of Medicine Committee on the Comprehensive Clinical Evaluation Program; the Presidential Advisory Committee on Gulf War Veterans' Illnesses; and a Veterans Administration Expert Panel) have conducted extensive reviews and published reports on the health of veterans and the possibility that they may have suffered adverse health effects as a result of some exposure during their period of service. The focus of these and other studies has been on assessing the current health of veterans, ensuring that appropriate care is being provided, and evaluating the possible connections between the current health status of veterans and their service in and specific exposures during the Gulf War. These expert panels have recommended improvements in U.S. Department of Defense (DoD) policies, procedures, and technologies for protecting the health of military personnel during deployments.

Deputy Secretary of Defense John White met with the leadership of the National Academies to discuss DoD's continuing efforts to improve its protection of military personnel from adverse health effects related to deployments in hostile environments. Although many of the lessons learned from previous assessments of Operation Desert Shield/Desert Storm have been reported, prospective analyses (1) to identify gaps and shortcomings in policy, doctrine, training, and equipment and (2) to develop a strategy to improve the management of battlefield health risks in future deployments have not been done. The DoD requested that the National Academies perform a prospective evaluation of strategies to protect deployed U.S. forces. This report, which addresses the issues of physical protection and decontamination, is one of four initial reports that will be submitted in response to that request.

CHARGE TO THE NATIONAL ACADEMIES

The DoD sought an independent, unbiased evaluation of the capabilities of current DoD research and development (R&D) in response to new threats, research priorities for filling important information and technology gaps, and recommendations for improving the effectiveness and responsiveness of R&D. The evaluations are focused on four areas: (1) risk assessments of deployments in hostile environments; (2) technologies and methods for detecting and tracking exposures to chemical agents, biological agents, and other harmful agents; (3) physical protection and decontamination; and (4) medical protection, health consequences and treatment, and medical record keeping. Studies addressing topics 1, 2, and 4 were conducted concurrently with this study by the Commission on Life Sciences, Commission on Engineering and Technical Systems, and the IOM, respectively.

Scope of the Study

The objective of this study, carried out under the auspices of the Commission on Engineering and Technical Systems, is to assess DoD's current and potential approaches and technologies for physical protection—both individual and collective—against CB agents and decontamination of personnel and equipment. The evaluation also examines the implementation of current policies, doctrine, and training as they relate to protection and decontamination of exposures to CB agents during troop deployments and recommends strategies to improve protection against deleterious health effects in future deployments. Specifically, this report includes a review and evaluation of the following areas:

- the adequacy of current protective equipment and protective measures (as well as equipment in development)
- the efficacy of current and proposed methods for decontaminating personnel and equipment after exposures to CB agents
- current policies, doctrine, and training to protect and decontaminate personnel and equipment in future deployments (i.e., major regional conflicts [MRCs], lesser regional conflicts [LRCs], and operations other than war [OOTWs])
- the impact of equipment and procedures on unit effectiveness and other human performance factors
- current and projected military capabilities to provide emergency response

Limitations

This report addresses nonmedical force protection (e.g., individual and collective protective clothing and equipment) in a potential CB environment. Medical aspects of nuclear, biological, and chemical (NBC) defense, including medical preventive measures (e.g., vaccines) and treatments (e.g., antidote kits) and their doctrine and training protocols, are addressed in the medical surveillance, record keeping, and risk reduction report (IOM, 1999a). The trade-offs between NBC medical defense and NBC nonmedical physical protection (e.g., protective clothing and masks) will be addressed in the third year study.

Radioactivity associated with nuclear weapons or other military uses of radioactive materials (i.e., depleted uranium) are not addressed in this report. Although individual and collective protective equipment is designed to protect against radioactive materials, this aspect of protection is beyond the scope of this study.

Since the end of the Cold War, multinational forces have been increasingly used in deployments. Coalition troops and U.S. troops should receive similar training and equipment and doctrine should be applied uniformly. However, this issue could not be evaluated in the present study because the data on doctrine and training are not sufficient. The authors encourage the North Atlantic Treaty Organization (NATO) to establish guidelines in these areas (e.g., NATO, 1996a, 1996b).

In keeping with the definition of deployment issued by the chairman of the JCS, this study does not explicitly consider the contamination of ships and other ocean vessels, even though they may be involved in the transportation of deploying forces and are potential CB targets. However, many aspects of personal protection, collective protection, and decontamination of land-based personnel and equipment may apply to shipboard situations. The contamination of aircraft personnel and equipment, as well as airfields, are included.

This study focuses only on deployed forces and does not explicitly consider nondeployed forces or nonmilitary contract employees who perform work in the host nation. Although these individuals are vital to successful missions and the technical aspects of protecting them may be the same as for deployed troops, the implementation of a protective strategy and the development of doctrine and training for them are beyond the scope of this study.

The shift to a Force Projection strategy and the decrease in the number of active duty personnel have increased U.S. dependence on Reserves and National Guard personnel. DoD has not yet developed a viable plan for preparing reserve forces for deployment in a CB environment. Their training may not be comparable to active-component training and their equipment may not be up to date. Nevertheless, the needs of the reserve units are the same as for active duty forces. (For a discussion of strategies for improving the integration of reserve components and active deployed forces see *Technology-Based Pilot Programs* [NRC, 1999a].)

APPROACH OF THE STUDY

The study was led by two principal investigators, an inhalation toxicologist with expertise in personal protection and a physical chemist with expertise in CB and military operations. A panel of advisors with expertise in respiratory protection, dermatology, systems engineering, human performance and human factors, and textiles provided additional support and advice.

The principal investigators and National Academies staff, with the participation of the advisory panel, made numerous site visits to DoD agencies and related organizations, hosted a series of public meetings and one public workshop, commissioned papers to address specific issues, attended demonstrations of current simulation and modeling efforts, and toured the facilities at the U.S. Army Chemical School, the Soldier and Biological Chemical Command (SBCCOM) Soldier Systems Center and the SBCCOM Edgewood Chemical Biological Center. In-depth briefings and presentations covered the following topics: the worldwide CB threat; the role and adequacy of threat information in materiel development from the perspectives of intelligence support and program managers; the method by which threat information is provided in response to research, development, test, and evaluation (RDT&E) questions; the way threat information is used to support the development of philosophy and doctrine; the relationship between physical protection and decontamination training protocols and doctrine; the consistency of training among Army components and among services; the way(s) threat information is used to support the development of physical protection and decontamination materiel; the status of current related programs and funding levels; and current and emerging technologies (including how they will address current and potential new threats). Additional sources of information included guidebooks, technical reports, field manuals, issue papers, information papers, journal articles, and information on the World Wide Web.

OVERVIEW OF THE REPORT

The remainder of this report is divided into seven chapters. Chapter 2 is an assessment of the threat and risk, including an historical overview of the development of CB agents and their use; a discussion of the theoretical relationships of policy, doctrine, training, R&D, and perceived threats; and the adequacy of threat information for the development of physical protection doctrine, training protocols, and materiel. Chapter 3 is a description of CB philosophy, doctrine, and training in light of the changing threat in the post-Cold War environment. In Chapter 4, physical protection, including protection levels; current and emerging technologies in fibers, textiles, and garments; respiratory protection; and training in the use of these technologies, are reviewed and assessed.

Decontamination is addressed in Chapter 5. Given the limitations of detection, monitoring, and providing protection, decontamination systems will always be necessary for personnel and equipment, as well as for nonpersonnel functional areas (e.g., sensitive equipment, facilities, large open areas). Because of their differing vulnerabilities and requirements, and because of the limitations of current decontamination systems, new technologies will have to be developed. Chapter 6 is a summary and assessment of methods of testing the elements of protective strategy and evaluating the effectiveness of training and readiness.

Chapter 7 provides a brief assessment of the military's capabilities to provide emergency response and references other work that specifically addresses this issue. The term "emergency response" in the CB arena refers to incidents of domestic terrorism, which is beyond the scope of this study. Nevertheless, the military plays a role in responding to CB domestic terrorism, CB terrorist attacks against U.S. facilities in other countries (e.g., U.S. embassies), and CB attacks against the military at U.S. points of embarkation.

Chapter 8 reviews and evaluates the relationship among R&D, funding, doctrine, and priorities; and summarizes the key findings and recommendations for continuing or beginning investments in various R&D areas. The discussion includes R&D in a joint service environment, changes brought about by new legislation, and the impact of laws and presidential directives on service programs. The chapter also includes key findings and priority recommendations for improving DoD's protection of deployed forces.

2

Threat and Risk Assessment

HISTORICAL PERSPECTIVE OF THE CHEMICAL/BIOLOGICAL BATTLE SPACE

CB agents have been considered effective weapons for combat for more than a millennium, from the tossing of plague victims over castle walls to the poisoning of water supplies and individuals. However, lethal CB weapons were first used extensively by the military in World War I (U.S. Army Office of the Surgeon General, 1997). Trench warfare, in which forces were deployed in fixed positions vulnerable to concentrated pockets of lethal fumes, provided fertile ground for the development of chemical weapons that could be dispersed as fogs, mists, or dense vapors. The first chemicals used during World War I were noxious gases (chlorine [Cl_2], hydrogen sulfide [H_2S], and phosgene [$COCl_2$]) and were released from upwind storage vessels along enemy lines. Local meteorological patterns were used to predict the movement of the gas clouds. However, this methodology was often ineffective because rapid changes could cause deadly clouds to settle on friendly forces, resulting in self-inflicted casualties. Early chemical agents were primarily inhalation threats, and effective gas masks (or respirators) were quickly developed and refined to protect personnel against toxic gases.

Respirators greatly diminished the tactical advantage of using toxic gases, and new chemical warfare agents had to be developed. Some of the new agents were chemical mustard agents, sulfur and nitrogen mustards, which caused serious injury and incapacitation not only when they were inhaled but also when they came into contact with the skin or mucous membranes. Because of the percutaneous threat of these agents, gas masks alone could no longer provide adequate protection, and garments to protect skin had to be developed.

In addition to new agents, new delivery systems were also developed. At first, artillery shells were modified to accommodate agents. Later, more sophisticated techniques evolved. Although there was still some risk that changes in local weather and climate could cause chemical agents to drift onto friendly targets, the risk was mitigated significantly as targeting became more accurate.

During the interval between World War I and World War II, new and more lethal families of chemical agents were developed. German scientists working to provide weapons for their military, discovered and refined a series of "nerve" agents—tabun (GA), soman (GD), and sarin (GB)—that attacked the central nervous system, could be absorbed through mucous membranes and the skin as well as inhaled, and were lethal in much smaller doses than the chemicals that had been used during World War I. At the same time, Japanese scientists were experimenting with agents of biological origin, such as plague and typhus. These agents were tested on human prisoners (U.S. Army Office of the Surgeon General, 1997).

Although neither chemical nor biological agents were actually used during World War II to achieve any military objectives, work continued and provided the foundation for the extensive CB research program of the Cold War powers. Led by scientists in the United States and the Soviet Union, the CB weapons programs flourished during the 1950s and 1960s. New nerve agents were developed (the family of V agents) that were not only more lethal in smaller inhaled doses but could also be absorbed directly through the skin. Existing agents were refined and mixed with additives to increase their persistence in the environment and the difficulty of decontamination.

During this time, natural toxins produced by biological organisms were also developed as weapons. The poisons produced, for example, by castor beans (ricin), puffer fish (tetrodotoxin), bacteria (botulinum), and fungi (mycotoxins) are among the most toxic compounds known and are lethal in even smaller quantities than V-agents. Although the production of large quantities of these toxins was difficult because of their high degree of lethality, much smaller amounts were required.

In addition to plague and typhus, other biological pathogens were studied as biological warfare agents, and weaponization techniques were researched and developed. Virtually every type of disease, condition, and means of dissemination was studied. From smallpox to cholera, from anthrax to hemorrhagic fevers, from tularemia to parasites, these agents and others were considered as possible weapons. The exposure of troops to pathogens or toxins through food supplies, water supplies, aerosols, and insect or animal vectors was also studied.

During the post-1950s era, the means of dissemination of lethal agents became major research objectives. Airborne spray tanks, specialized artillery shells, CB-capable missile warheads, and an assortment of individual weapons were developed. At the same time, the threat of exposure led to the development of defenses. Protection (both individual and collective) and decontamination became high-priority issues and stimulated the development of protective equipment. Thus, gas masks, protective garments, boots, gloves, protective shelters, and decontaminating solutions and systems were produced.

Even as the development of more and more lethal agents continued, societal fears and the conviction that the use of weapons of mass destruction was unethical resulted in treaties and international agreements that limited the proliferation, control, and testing of CB weapons. The Geneva Protocol of 1925 condemned the use in war of asphyxiating, poisonous, or other gases, as well as bacteriological warfare. The United States signed the Geneva Protocol but did not ratify it until 1975. However, the United States reserved the right not to be bound by the protocol if any enemy or state or any of its allies did not respect the protocol.

In 1972, the Biological and Toxins Weapons Convention (BWC) was signed. Under the terms of the convention, the parties agreed not to develop, produce, stockpile, or acquire biological agents, toxins, weapons, or means of delivery. Many years later, the Chemical Weapons Convention (CWC) banned the acquisition, development, production, transfer, and use of chemical weapons throughout the world. The United States signed the CWC in 1993 but did not ratify it until 1997. On June 25, 1999, the President issued an Executive Order implementing the CWC; it went into effect on June 26, 1999.

Since the implementation of these treaties, both the United States and the former Soviet Union have embarked on programs to destroy residual stockpiles (U.S. Army Office of the Surgeon General, 1997). However, CB technologies have been transferred to, and proliferated in, other countries; and modern bioengineering and molecular biological capabilities have given even small nations and groups the capability of developing novel, lethal agents. Documentation of the use of chemical weapons in localized wars and credible warnings from the intelligence community confirm that many potential enemies in regions to which U.S. forces may be deployed have the capability of using CB weapons.

Thus, the United States could find itself confronted with adversaries who have either chosen not to sign and ratify the CWC and/or BWC or have chosen to ignore them. Nevertheless, as a signatory of both the CWC and BWC, the United States has adopted a national policy of not using biological or chemical weapons in warfare even in retaliation for a CB attack. This asymmetrical threat has led to a national military strategy based on defense and deterrence (Chow et al., 1998; DoD, 1995; Joint Chiefs of Staff, 1995; Secretary of Defense, 1999; U.S. Army and U.S. Marine Corps, 1996). The policy is to deter the use of CB agents by enabling U.S. forces to survive, fight, and win a war under CB conditions. This policy has stimulated a continuing research program for refining military doctrine, for developing protective technologies, and for training U.S. forces against CB attack.

U.S. RESPONSE

The Army Chemical Corps has historically been the military organization primarily responsible for dealing with CB threats. Founded in June 1918 as the Chemical Warfare Service and renamed the Army Chemical Corps in August 1946, the Army Chemical Corps has alternately enjoyed support and been threatened with elimination, depending on political and economic exigencies. Prior to 1920, the development of chemical defenses was not tightly structured. Various chemical warfare schools (called gas schools) existed, but no single department was responsible for coordinating chemical warfare activities. The Army assumed the *de facto* role of executive agent for CB R&D by virtue of its large and long-term investment in the development of chemical equipment and its extensive experience with chemical exposure on the battlefield. The Army controlled the production of chemicals, the development and production of defensive equipment, training, testing, basic research, and a new chemical warfare unit.

Although the Army was more actively involved in this area than other services, in fact each military service was free to develop its own CB defense program and materiel. Each service had a separate budget and administered the budget and its program independently, cooperating with other services as the needs of basic or developmental research dictated. Each service also prioritized its needs for equipment separately, on the basis of service-specific needs. As operations became more and more integrated and cooperative (joint operations), both Congress and the military departments recognized the need for joint R&D programs and integrated procedures to improve joint operations and decrease logistical support burdens. This need has become more compelling as budgets have become more constrained and the cost of duplication of equipment has become unsupportable.

In the early 1990s, Congress began to encourage joint R&D programs. However, encouragement was not enough to overcome decades of independent activities (Nilo, 1999). Therefore, Congress passed Public Law

(PL) 103-160, the National Defense Authorization Act for Fiscal Year 1994 (Title XVII), which included the following stipulations (U.S. Congress, 1994):

- The CB defense program would be coordinated by a single DoD office that would oversee the program through the Defense Acquisition Board process.
- The CB defense program would have a coordinated/integrated budget.
- CB defense funds would be administered from DoD-level accounts.
- The Army would be the executive agent for coordination and integration of the CB defense program.

In order to meet the requirements of PL 103-160, a new structure, the Joint NBC[1] Defense Board, was established to provide oversight and management of DoD's NBC defense program (Figure 2-1). The NBC Defense Board's responsibilities include approval of (1) joint NBC requirements; (2) the Joint NBC Modernization Plan; (3) the consolidated NBC Defense Program Objective Memorandum (POM); (4) the Joint NBC Research, Development, and Acquisition (RDA) Plan; (5) joint training and doctrine initiatives; and (6) the Joint NBC Logistics Support Plan. The Joint NBC Defense Board Secretariat is responsible for management of program and acquisition strategies; planning, programming, budgeting, and execution of the program; and consolidation and integration of CB requirements and programs for all services.

Two subordinate groups support the Joint NBC Defense Board: the Joint Service Integration Group (JSIG) and the Joint Service Materiel Group (JSMG). The JSIG is responsible for joint NBC requirements, priorities, training, and doctrine. Thus, the JSIG develops a prioritized list of needs, requirements, and programs, which are based on commander-in-chief (CINC) priorities, threat projections, and analyses. A list of current, integrated CINC priorities, as well as the NBC Defense Program priorities can be found in Tables 2-1 and 2-2.

The priorities identified by the JSIG are inputs to the JSMG, which is responsible for the coordination, integration, planning, and programming of nonmedical RDA, science and technology, and logistics sustainment. Other responsibilities of the JSMG include preparation of the Joint Service NBC Defense RDA Plan, preparation of the Joint Service NBC Defense Logistics Support Plan, continuous review of the technology base, and reviews of developmental programs for possible NBC defense applications

---

[1]Although the NBC defense program addresses nuclear, as well as chemical and biological threats, the National Academies was only asked to address chemical and biological threats. Thus, this report only includes the chemical and biological aspects of CB defense.

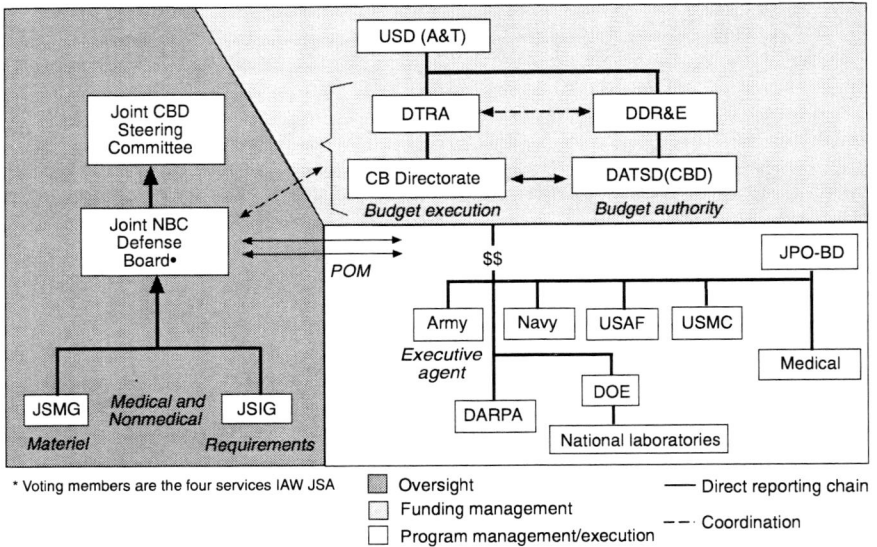

FIGURE 2-1 Management structure of the DoD Chemical and Biological Defense Program

Note: CBD = chemical/biological defense; DARPA = Defense Advanced Research Projects Agency; DATSD (CBD) = Deputy Assistant to the Secretary of Defense for Chemical/Biological Defense; DDR&E = Director, Defense Research and Engineering; DOE = U.S. Department of Energy; DTRA = Defense Threat Reduction Agency; IAW JSA = in accordance with the joint service agreement; JPO-BD = Joint Program Office for Biological Defense; JSIG = Joint Service Integration Group; JSMG = Joint Service Materiel Group; USAF = United States Air Force; USD(A&T) = Undersecretary of Defense (Acquisition and Technology); USMC = U.S. Marine Corps

Source: Nilo, 1999.

and/or impacts. The JSMG and the JSIG jointly prepare the consolidated NBC Defense POM strategy.

The services receive funding for NBC defense programs from the Office of the Secretary of Defense after having their inputs considered by the NBC Defense Board. Programmatic and other decisions are based on a formal voting process in which each member has one vote. The membership of each group (the NBC Defense Board, the JSIG, and the JSMG) consists of representatives of each of the services, the joint staff, the Defense Logistics Agency, the Joint Program Office for Biological Defense (JPO-BD), the Medical Research Materiel Command, and the Special Operations Command.

TABLE 2-1 Integrated CINC Priorities

1.	Intelligence
2.	Precision attack with no collateral damage
3.	Special operations forces counterterrorism
4.	NBC detection and warning
5.	Theater missile defense with no collateral damage
6.	Defeat underground targets
7.	Target planning and battle damage assessment
8.	Individual protection
9.	Proliferation pathway analysis
10.	Cruise missile DEF/ADA with no collateral damage
11.	Collective protection
12.	Defeat mobile target
13.	Offensive information warfare
14.	Logistics consequences capability
15.	Decontamination
16.	NBC medical treatment

Source: Nilo, 1999.

Execution of the RDA program under the JSMG is controlled by a group of five commodity area managers. Each service has been assigned lead responsibility for the commodity area most closely aligned with its expertise: contamination avoidance—Army; individual protection—Marine Corps; collective protection—Navy; decontamination—Air Force; medical protection—Medical Research Materiel Command. These commodity area managers are responsible for developing materiel that is usable in the field.

Discussions with personnel at the U.S. Army Chemical School, Soldier and Biological Chemical Command, JSMG, Deputy Chief of Staff for Operations, and outside contractors revealed general dissatisfaction with the prioritization process because service-specific projects were often given priority over projects based on multiservice needs through a process of political compromise and CINC priorities were largely ignored in the process (Blankenbiller, 1998; Nilo, 1999; U.S. Army SBCCOM, 1998). A comparison of CINC priorities (shown in Table 2-1) and program priorities (shown in Table 2-2) lends some credence to these complaints.

RELATIONSHIPS AMONG POLICY; DOCTRINE; RESEARCH, DEVELOPMENT AND ACQUISITION; AND THREAT

The intelligence community provides data, analysis, and advice on the development of CB capabilities of threat nations. Based on information about the types, quantities, and delivery systems of CB agents, CINCs and the JSIG evaluate the ways these agents could be used against U.S.

TABLE 2-2 Nuclear, Biological, Chemical (NBC) Nonmedical Defense Program Priorities

Priority	Area	Program
1	CA	Joint Biological Point Detection System
2	CA	Joint Biological Remote Early Warning System
3	CA	Joint Service Light NBC Reconnaissance System
4	BM	Joint Warning and Reporting Network
5	CA	Joint Service Lightweight Standoff Chemical Agent Detector
6	CA	Biological Integrated Detection Systems
7	CA	Chemical/Biological Mass Spectrometer
8	CA	Interim Biological Agent Detector
9	IP	Joint Lightweight Integrated Suit Technology (JLIST)
10	CA	Joint Chemical Agent Detector
11	IP	Aircrew Mask Programs
12	CA	NBC Reconnaissance System Product Improvement Program
13	CA	Automatic Chemical Agent Detector and Alarm
14	RES	Joint Service Fixed-Site Decontamination
15	CA	Long-Range Biological Stand-off Detection System
16	IP	Protection Assessment Test System
17	RES	Joint Service Sensitive Equipment Decontamination
18	IP	M40A1 Series Mask
19	CA	Special Operations Modular Chemical/Biological Detector
20	IP	Joint Service Aviation Mask
21	CA	Joint Service Warning and Identification LIDAR Detector
22	IP	Joint Protective Aircrew Chemical Ensemble
23	IP	Chemical Environment Survivability Suit
24	RES	Fixed-Site Decontamination Subitem: Joint Advanced Decontamination System
25	CP	Joint Transportable Collective Protection System
26	BM	Multipurpose Integrated Chemical Agent Alarm
27	CA	Shipboard Automatic Agent Detector
28	CA	Improved Chemical Agent Monitor
29	CP	Shipboard Collective Protective Equipment
30	CA	Improved Point Detection System
31	IP	Joint Service General Purpose Mask
32	CP	Joint Collective Protection Improvement Program
33	RES	Joint Lightweight Portable Decontamination System
34	CA	Joint Chemical/Biological Agent Water Monitor
35	RES	Lightweight Decontamination System
36	RES	Modular Decontamination System
37	RES	Sorbent Decontamination System
38	IP	Joint Canteen Refilling System
39	IP	Chemical Environment Survivability Mask
40	CA	Pocket RADIAC (Radioactivity, Detection, Indication, and Computation)
41	CP	Advanced Integrated Collective Protection System
42	CA	NBC Unmanned Ground Vehicle Sensor
43	CA	Stand-off RADIAC
44	CA	Advanced Airborne RADIAC System

CA = contamination avoidance; BM = battle space management; IP = individual protection (also known as personal protection); RES = restoration (decontamination); CP = collective protection
Source: Nilo, 1999.

troops. Their evaluation is then used to develop policy, doctrine, training, and equipment to counter the perceived threat. As the threat changes, approaches to countering the threat should also change.

The mission to protect forces from the effects of CB weapons has developed into a five-pronged approach. The thrust of current doctrine is to avoid contamination/exposure and to prevent adverse health effects. Three major elements of this approach (individual protection, collective protection, and decontamination) will be discussed in detail in subsequent sections of this report.[2]

Contamination Avoidance

Prior to deployment, the intelligence community provides up-to-date assessments of the potential threat of the use of CB agents to achieve military objectives. This assessment is critical to determining the types of detection equipment, protective equipment, and CB specialists that will be necessary for the deployment. State-of-the-art detector systems, both stand-off and local monitors, can identify potential threats in advance to enable commanders to avoid areas of contamination or to take protective measures to avoid exposures. Detectors can also be used to evaluate levels of contamination so commanders can select appropriate protection for their forces and minimize the length of time spent in protective clothing. The report of Task 2.2 assesses technologies and methods for detecting, tracking, and monitoring exposures of deployed U.S. forces to potentially harmful agents, including, chemical and biological agents and environmental contaminants (NRC, 1999b).

Individual Protection

Individuals can be protected by individual protective equipment (breathing masks with high-efficiency filters that selectively remove noxious agents, chemically treated clothing that can prevent agents from contacting the skin, and gloves and boot covers that are impervious to noxious agents) if they have been properly trained in rapidly donning the equipment and removing contaminated equipment safely, and if they receive adequate warning. Commanders need appropriate doctrine to establish the level of protection to minimize the risk to troops while allowing them to complete their mission.

---

[2]Contamination avoidance and medical systems are the subjects of separate detailed reports (IOM, 1999a; NRC, 1999b).

Collective Protection

Collective protection provides a contamination-free area (e.g., passenger compartments of military vehicles, shelters) for eating, rest, and relief from the constraints of individual protective equipment. It also provides a safe working environment for command and control functions and can be used for medical treatment of casualties in the CB environment.

Decontamination

Decontamination may be necessary for equipment and personnel before they can be returned to combat. Decontamination may also be necessary to restore mission-critical assets to operational status. Large-scale decontamination of major resources (e.g., airfields or buildings) may be necessary to support embarkation/debarkation phases of a deployment.

Medical Systems

Medical systems provide predeployment and postexposure treatment for CB-induced health problems and maintain records on health and exposures for deployed personnel. The development of antibodies, vaccines, and medical therapies is a critical part of the medical systems.

CHARACTERISTICS OF CURRENT AND FUTURE CHEMICAL AND BIOLOGICAL AGENTS

Effects and Tactical Utility of Chemical Agents

Chemical agents can be characterized as either lethal or nonlethal (incapacitating) (see Table 2-3); however, these distinctions have more to do with intent and use than with the composition of the agents because all agents are lethal in high concentrations. There are three classifications of lethal agents: nerve agents, choking agents, and blood agents.

Nerve agents inhibit acetylcholinesterase, an enzyme involved in the transmission of nerve impulses. Inhibition of this enzyme results in continuous stimulation of the nervous system. Nerve agents act more quickly and are more lethal than other chemical agents. They can be absorbed through the skin, the eyes, or the respiratory tract. Symptoms include runny nose, tightness in the chest, impaired vision, pinpointing of the pupils, difficulty in breathing, excessive salivation and drooling, nausea, vomiting, cramps, involuntary twitching, loss of bowel and bladder control, headache, confusion, drowsiness, coma, and eventually death.

Choking agents, which are primarily taken in via the respiratory tract,

TABLE 2-3 Categorization of Chemical Agents

Type	Examples
Lethal Chemical Agents	
Blood agents	hydrogen cyanide, cyanogen chloride, arsine
Choking agents	phosgene, diphosgene, chlorine
Nerve agents	tabun, sarin, soman, GF, VX
Incapacitating Chemical Agents	
Blister agents (vesicants)	Levinstein mustard, distilled mustard, nitrogen mustard, mustard-t mixture, lewisite, mustard-lewisite mixture, phenyldichloroarsine, ethyldichloroarsine, methyldichloroarsine, phosgene oxime
Lacrimator agents	bromobenzylcyanide, chloroacetophenone, CNC, o-chlorobenzylidene malononitrile, dibenz-(b,f)-1,4-oxazepine, chloropicrin
Sternutator agents	diphenylchloroarsine, diphenylcyanoarsine, adamsite

are strong irritants that attack lung tissues causing membranes to swell and become "leaky." The lung can then fill with fluid, and death can result from pulmonary edema. Acute nonlethal exposures to choking agents can result in chronic lung disease.

Blood agents are primarily absorbed via the respiratory tract. They inhibit the enzyme cytochrome oxidase or combine with hemoglobin to prevent the normal transfer of oxygen from the blood to body tissues. Exposure to these agents causes seizures due to lack of oxygenation.

Agents classified as nonlethal or incapacitating include vesicants, lacrimators, and sternutators. Vesicants, or blister agents, which affect the eyes and lungs and blister the skin, are often lethal if ingested or absorbed through the lungs. Lacrimators cause tearing and irritate the skin and respiratory tract. Sternutators cause coughing, nausea, and vomiting.

An agent's tactical utility is partly determined by its physical properties including: (1) whether the agent is effective in the short or long term (persistence of the agent in the environment); (2) whether the agent can be targeted to a specific area or is affected by wind and weather conditions; (3) whether the agent presents an inhalation or percutaneous threat, or both; (4) whether the agent is stable during dissemination; and (5) other physical and chemical factors.

Agents are often characterized as persistent (lasting longer than 24 hours as a hazard) or nonpersistent (lasting less than 24 hours as a hazard). Ordinarily, persistent agents are disseminated as liquids, and nonpersistent agents are disseminated as gases. However, most agents, through the use of additives, can be made persistent or nonpersistent.

The actual use of CB weapons may not be necessary because the threat of CB weapons may result in troops taking defensive measures. Forces threatened by CB weapons will be burdened by the need to transport protective gear and decontamination equipment, and the effectiveness of fighting units can be diminished if personnel are forced to operate in protective gear. The threat of CB weapons will also increase the psychological burden of personnel.

Effects and Tactical Utility of Biological Agents

Biological agents can be classified into three main groups: pathogenic microorganisms, viruses, and toxins. The first two groups are living, self-replicating organisms; however, viruses only self-replicate in a host. Toxins are poisons (nonliving) produced by bacteria, plants, or fungi. Table 2-4 gives examples for each category of biological warfare agents.

Pathogenic microorganisms can be classified as protozoa, fungi, bacteria, and rickettsia. Protozoa are one-celled organisms that are motile. Fungi are organisms that do not use photosynthesis, are capable of anaerobic growth, and draw nutrition from decaying vegetable matter. Most fungi form spores.

Because bacteria are much better understood than other biological agents, they are the most likely type of biological warfare agents (Ali et al., 1997). Bacteria are small free-living organisms, most of which can be grown on a solid or in a liquid culture. Bacterial structures consist of nuclear material, cytoplasm, and cell membranes. They vary in shape and size from spherical cells and cocci (with a diameter of 0.5 to 1.0 microns) to bacilli (with a diameter of 1.0 to 5.0 microns). In response to changes in their environment, some types of bacteria can change into spores, which are more resistant to cold, heat, drying, chemicals, and radiation, than bacteria themselves. Diseases caused by bacteria often respond to treatment with antibiotics.

Viruses vary in size from 0.02 to 0.2 microns and must be cultivated in living cells in order to multiply. Rickettsiae have characteristics common to both bacteria and viruses. They resemble bacteria in that they possess metabolic enzymes and cell membranes, utilize oxygen, and are susceptible to antibiotics. They are similar to viruses in that they only grow in living cells.

TABLE 2-4 Categorization of Biological Agents

Type	Examples
Pathogenic Biological Agents	
Protozoa	malaria
Bacteria	*Bacillus anthracis, Yersinia pestis, Francisella tularensis, Shigella dysenteriae, Vibrio comma, Brucella suis, Salmonella typhimurium, Shigella dysenteriae*
Rickettsiae	*Coxiella burneti, Rickettsia rickettsia*
Fungi	coccidioides immitis
Viruses	smallpox, Venezuelan equine encephalitis, yellow fever, Rift Valley fever
Toxins	
Bacterial toxins	botulinum toxin, *Clostridium perfringens* toxin, staphylococcus enterotoxin B
Plant toxins	ricin
Fungal toxins	T-2 mycotoxins

There are three classifications of toxins: plant toxins, bacterial toxins, and fungal toxins. Plant toxins, poisons that are naturally produced by plants, are easy to acquire in large quantities at minimal cost in a low-technology environment. Bacterial toxins, poisons that are naturally produced through the metabolic activities of bacteria, are harder to produce on a large scale than plant toxins, but they are many times more toxic. Fungal toxins, which are produced by various species of fungi, are much less toxic than bacterial and plant toxins in vapor form, but unlike the other toxins they are dermally active.

The tactical utility of biological agents depends on their robustness, their dissemination characteristics, their persistence (see Box 2-1), their ability to multiply and cause infections, and other factors. There are effective means for protection (e.g., antibodies and vaccines) against some biological warfare agents; however, nations that do not adhere to the BWC and CWC are constantly attempting to modify agents to defeat conventional defenses.

> **BOX 2-1 Persistence of Biological Agents**
>
> **Anthrax.** Spores are very stable but will be destroyed in a matter of hours by sunlight. The vegetative form is very unstable. Spores remain alive in soil and water for many years. Spores can be killed by dry heat at >284°F for one hour, boiling contaminated items in water for 30 minutes or more, or by treating with heat or certain acids (i.e., perchloric acid) or alkalies (i.e., sodium hypochlorite).
>
> ***Yersinia pestis*** **(plague).** Not very hearty once released into the environment but stable and viable in water from 2–30 days and in moist soil for about two weeks. At near freezing temperatures, it will remain alive for years. It can be killed by exposure to heat at 130°F for 15 minutes, steam, three to five hours in sunlight, Lysol, or lime.
>
> ***Francisella tularensis*** **(tularemia).** Not extremely stable when released into the environment but remains viable for weeks in water, soil, carcasses, fur, and hides. In the frozen state, it is viable for years. It can be killed by heat at 113°F for a few minutes or by 0.5 percent phenol in 15 minutes.
>
> ***Shigella dysentariae*** **(dysentery).** Viable for a considerable period in water, ice, and mucous membranes but can be killed by sunlight, steam sterilization, and common disinfectants.
>
> ***Coxiella burneti*** **(Q fever).** Very stable and can remain active on surfaces for up to 60 days or in soils for months. It can be killed by 0.5 percent formalin.
>
> ***Vibrio comma*** **(cholera).** Will not remain viable in pure water and is unstable in aerosols but will survive up to 24 hours in raw sewage and six weeks in certain types of impure water containing salt and organic matter. Can be killed by drying.
>
> ***Rickettsia rickettsia*** **(Rocky Mountain spotted fever).** Can be killed by exposure to a temperature of 112°F for 10 minutes and by drying for 10 hours. Is deactivated by 0.1 percent formalin or 0.5 percent phenol.
>
> ***Brucella suis*** **(brucellosis).** Will remain alive for weeks in water, unpasteurized dairy products, and soil, but does not survive long when airborne. Common methods of sterilization or disinfection will kill the organism.

PROLIFERATION OF CHEMICAL AND BIOLOGICAL AGENTS

Both open literature and intelligence assessments indicate that many nations are attempting to develop chemical, and possibly biological, weapons. Although the number of countries that possess CB capabilities is troubling, intelligence assessments also indicate that most of these countries have limited quantities of agents and limited delivery systems. Estimates also indicate that most proliferant countries have neither the industrial infrastructure nor the military logistics capabilities to produce chemical weapons in sufficient quantity to pose an extensive threat to

Salmonella typhimurium. Stable for up to two weeks in water, up to three months in ice and snow, and one to two months in feces. Exposure to heat at 132°F for 20 minutes or exposure for five minutes to 5 percent phenol or bichloride of mercury will kill it.

Smallpox. Highly stable and retains its infectivity for long periods outside the host. Decontamination can be accomplished by exposure of the organism to alcohol and acetone for one hour at room temperature or by exposure to chlorine. Moist heat above 140°F and dry heat above 212°F will also decontaminate the organism.

Venezuelan equine encephalitis. Relatively unstable. Standard decontaminants and methods will sterilize the agent.

Yellow fever. Relatively unstable.

Botulism. Nonpersistent and stable for 12 hours in air, seven days in solution when protected from light and heat, and longer in food not exposed to air. Boiling for 15 minutes or cooking food for 30 minutes at 175°F destroys it.

Staphylococcus enterotoxin B. Nonpersistent but stable in heat and acid and alkali solutions. Resistant to freezing and boiling for 30 minutes. The organism that develops the toxin remains viable after 67 days of refrigeration. Formaldehyde detoxifies it.

Clostridium perfringens. Purified toxin is relatively unstable and very sensitive to heat.

Ricin. Persistent and stable in water or dilute acid. Weak hypochlorite solutions, chlorine, or soap and water will sterilize the organism.

Sources: U.S. Army et al., 1990; U.S. Army, 1995; U.S. Air Force, 1997; Boyle, 1998a.

troops with adequate protective capabilities. These countries are, however, capable of producing chemical weapons that can threaten unprotected or minimally protected forces and fixed sites, can be used in terrorist operations, or can be used as deterrents (Commission to Assess the Organization of the Federal Government to Combat the Proliferation of Weapons of Mass Destruction, 1999). Current assessments also indicate that these nations are not likely to possess novel chemical agents or to have weaponized biological agents. Thus, current U.S. protective approaches are likely to be effective.

Intelligence reports suggest that several agents may be in the process of development or weaponization in various countries. With recent advances in biomolecular engineering methods, existing pathogens can be modified to increase their toxicity or to defeat available defensive measures (i.e., vaccines). In fact, biomolecular engineering methods can also be used to modify (i.e., mutate) nonpathogenic organisms into disease-causing agents, thus increasing the potential of biological warfare threats. Because of the rapid developments in molecular biology, the spectrum of biological agents will continue to change, and protective measures will have to be continuously adjusted. Although a detailed review of these developments is beyond the scope of this study (for more information see Ali et al., 1997; DoD, 1996; Rose, In press), they should be kept in mind because they greatly complicate contamination avoidance.

Thickened and dusty agents have been areas of intense research, but the capacity for weaponizing these agents is, as yet, limited. New stabilizing agents have been developed that increase the persistence of a chemical agent and impede decontamination under some conditions. These stabilizers can allow degradation products to recombine into toxic forms at a later time, increasing their potential to affect areas contacted by runoff from decontamination (Ali et al., 1997).

The descriptions of threats posed by proliferant nations sharply contrast the descriptions for the former Soviet Union. Most proliferant countries do not have the research or industrial base to build a large-scale military capability that could threaten deployed U.S. forces, much less the logistical infrastructure to maintain a battlefield capability. However, the threat description on which U.S. requirements are based has changed very little (Eck, 1998).

PRODUCTION, WEAPONIZATION, AND DISPERSION

Military organizations worldwide have been working on the weaponization of CB agents. Chemical agents engineered for stability can be delivered from spray tanks, artillery shells, or missile warheads. They can also be introduced directly into food supplies, water supplies, and air-handling systems. Ordinarily, biological agents are much more environmentally sensitive than chemical agents and lose their effectiveness quickly when exposed to the atmosphere, and spreading most biological warfare agents from one infected individual to another (with the exception of smallpox) is difficult. The weaponization of biological agents can also be much more difficult than the weaponization of chemical agents (anthrax spores are an obvious exception).

The weaponization of chemical agents, thus far, has been limited to known delivery systems; and current proliferant nations are not likely to have delivery capabilities equal to the capability of the Soviet Union during the Cold War. Thus, even if chemical agents are transferred from a producing country to a nonproducing proliferant nation, the probability of transferring sufficient quantities to threaten massed U.S. forces is low. However, many countries could deploy sufficient amounts of CB weapons to threaten fixed sites and small units (Chow et al., 1998).

THREATENED USE OF CHEMICAL AND BIOLOGICAL WEAPONS

Proliferant nations could use CB weapons for several purposes: battlefield use against neighboring countries with similar military capabilities; battlefield use against U.S. or other asymmetrically powerful forces; as a weapon of terror; or as a means of changing public opinion. Because of logistical limitations and U.S. capabilities, widespread battlefield use against U.S. forces by nations currently known to have CB capabilities seems unlikely. However, the use of CB agents against neighboring countries or as a terrorist weapon against U.S. forces (especially forces occupying fixed sites) or U.S. peacekeeping teams is a legitimate threat.

Understanding the conditions under which an enemy might use CB weapons is central to the U.S. response. Adversaries in regional conflicts may have very different ideas than Cold War adversaries. For example, they may use CB weapons early in a conflict for political and psychological, as well as military, purposes (Joseph, 1996).

ASSESSMENT OF CHEMICAL AND BIOLOGICAL WARFARE RISKS

The threat to U.S. forces can be defined as the capability attributed to an opposing force. The risk for U.S. forces is determined through an analysis of the potential interactions of opposing forces. The decision to assume a protective posture is based on several factors, which are parallel to factors in other areas of risk assessment/risk management. The first stage in any risk assessment is hazard identification. In the context of this study, hazard identification requires evaluating the biomedical effects of individual agents on humans. The next stage is threat assessment, which requires determining the capability of an opponent to mount a CB attack and assessing the opponent's intent. The last step is to assess the probability of exposure for deployed forces and assess their ability to protect themselves. Having assessed the risk, one can then develop an approach to managing that risk.

Hazards: Routes and Levels of Exposure

Agents do not pose a hazard to humans until they are introduced into the body through the respiratory tract, the gastrointestinal tract, the mucous membranes, or the skin. The routes of effective exposure for various agents are described in the following Tables 2-5 through 2-11.

Effects of Chemical Agents

Inhalation/Respiratory Agents. Chemical agents that present inhalation/respiratory hazards are delivered as vapors or aerosols. An aerosol is defined as a particle (either liquid or solid) suspended in a gas (air). The particles in an aerosol, over time, will be removed from the air and deposited on the ground, on equipment, or on personnel by gravity, inertial impaction, or diffusion. The duration of time a particle can remain airborne and the distance a particle can travel depend on wind, humidity, particle size, and the height at which the particle is introduced into the air.

Vapors can form mixtures with air and can travel over great distances. Because vapors diffuse readily into the air, their concentration tends to decrease over time. Vapors can be removed from the air by diffusion to solid or liquid surfaces or by incorporation on, or in, airborne particles. The effects of inhaled agents are generally proportional to the amount inhaled (dose). For the purposes of this discussion, the effects are considered to be cumulative (a reasonable assumption because these agents are acutely toxic and exert their effects over relatively short time intervals). The dosages are presented in terms of concentration × time (Ct). Thus, an exposure to an agent at a concentration of 30 mg/m^3 for a period of 60 minutes would produce a dose of 1,800 mg-min/m^3 (see Table 2-5). The dose that was incapacitating to 50 percent of a given population (ID_{50}), the Ct dose that was incapacitating to 50 percent of a given population (ICt_{50}), and the Ct dose that caused the defined effect (e.g., edema or death) in 50 percent of a given population (ECt_{50}) are presented in units of mg-min/m^3.

Dermal Absorption Agents. Agents that are delivered as liquids or droplet aerosols can be absorbed through the skin (percutaneous absorption). Most of the nerve agents in liquid or vapor phase and many of the vesicants can be absorbed percutaneously. Thus, many chemical agents can present a hazard even if personnel are wearing respirators. Chemical agents that can be taken up percutaneously are described in Table 2-6.

Dermal Necrotic Agents. Blister agents can kill or destroy skin cells causing severe chemical burns. Lewisite causes painful injuries almost immediately upon exposure. Sulfur and nitrogen mustards have a delayed reaction and, therefore, have more insidious effects that may not occur for hours after exposure. The actual delay depends on the intensity of exposure and the area of skin exposed. Dermal necrotic agents are summarized in Table 2-7.

Ocular Agents. Many agents that cause inhalation/respiratory effects are also toxic to the eye, especially vesicant agents, such as sulfur mustard (HD). Available data indicate that temporary blindness could be produced by HD vapor exposures of 200 mg-min/m^3. Both GD and GB are known to have ocular effects, but the data are insufficient to establish an ECt_{50} (although GD is 2.5 times more potent as a meiotic agent than GB). The data on ocular effects are included in Tables 2-6 and 2-7.

Ingestion/Gastrointestinal Agents. Both food and water sources can become contaminated during an attack, but very little data are available on the effects after ingestion by humans, and information on animal models is spotty at best. At the present time, few methods are available for the rapid detection of chemical agents in either food or water. Toxic effects following ingestion will probably be similar to those after inhalation or percutaneous absorption.

Effects of Biological Agents

Inhalation/Respiratory Agents. Biological agents can be dispersed as aerosols and inhaled. The number of organisms or spores that represent an effective dose for agents known to be distributed in airborne form are summarized in Table 2-8 along with the expected effects and approximate time of onset of effects. The intensity of the exposure could alter the effect and the time to onset.

Ingestion/Gastrointestinal Agents. Biological agents can be ingested by hand-to-mouth activities or by the consumption of contaminated food or water. The contamination of foodstuffs can be deliberate or can occur as the result of environmental contamination from a more general attack using airborne agents. Information on ingestion and gastrointestinal agents is summarized in Table 2-9.

Percutaneous/Mucous Membrane Agents. The eyes are poorly defended both physically and physiologically and therefore represent a potential route of entry for pathogens. Other mucous membranes are also vulnerable to many agents. The biological agents associated with percutaneous and mucous membrane absorption are listed in Table 2-10.

TABLE 2-5 Inhalation/Respiratory Agents

Agent	Mode of Delivery	Effect
Phosgene	Vapor	Causes fluid buildup in the lungs that can cause drowning
Diphosgene	Vapor	Causes fluid buildup in the lungs that can cause drowning
Tabun	Vapor	Cessation of breath
Sarin	Vapor	Incapacitation; cessation of breath
Soman	Vapor	Incapacitation; cessation of breath
GF	Vapor	Incapacitation; cessation of breath
VX	Vapor	Incapacitation; cessation of breath
Hydrogen cyanide	Vapor	Interferes with the body's utilization of oxygen; accelerates rate of breathing

THREAT AND RISK ASSESSMENT

Effective Dose (mg-min/m³ except where otherwise noted)	Rate of Action
$ICt_{50} = 1{,}600$	Delayed, although immediate irritation in high concentrations. At low concentrations, no effects for three hours or more
$ICt_{50} = 1{,}600$ (at rest)	Delayed, although immediate irritation in high concentrations. At low concentrations, no effects for three hours or more
$ICt_{50} = 300$ (at rest) $Ect_{50} = $ no existing estimates $Ect_{50} = $ no existing estimates (severe effects)[a] $Ect_{50} = 0.9$ (mild effects)[a] $Ect_{50} = 2\text{--}3$[b]	Very rapid
$ICt_{50} = 75$ (at rest); 35 (mildly active) $ECt_{50} = $ no existing estimates (threshold)[a] $ECt_{50} = 35$ (severe effects)[a] $ECt_{50} = 2$ (mild effects)[a] $ECt_{50} = 3$[b]	Very rapid
$ICt_{50} = 75\text{--}300$ (at rest) $ECt_{50} = $ no existing estimates (threshold)[a] $ECt_{50} = 35$ (severe effects)[a] $ECt_{50} = $ no existing estimates (mild effects)[a] $ECt_{50} = 1\text{--}2$[b]	Very rapid
$ECt_{50} = $ no existing estimates (threshold) $ECt_{50} = $ no existing estimates (severe effects) $ECt_{50} = $ no existing estimates (mild effects)	Very rapid
$ICt_{50} = 50$ (at rest); 24 (mildly active) $ECt_{50} = $ no existing estimates (threshold)[a] $ECt_{50} = 25$ (severe effects)[a] $ECt_{50} = 0.09$ (mild effects)[a] $ECt_{50} = 1\text{--}2$[b]	Very rapid
ICt_{50} varies with concentration $ECt_{50} = \sim 1{,}500$	Very rapid; incapacitation can occur within 1 to 2 minutes of exposure to an incapacitating or lethal dose, and death can occur within 15 minutes of receiving a lethal dose

TABLE 2-5 Inhalation/Respiratory Agents (continued)

Agent	Mode of Delivery	Effect
Cyanogen chloride	Vapor	Choking, irritation, slows breathing
Arsine	Vapor	Damages blood, liver, and kidneys
Distilled mustard	Vapor	Inflammation of the nose, throat, trachea, bronchi, and lungs
Nitrogen mustard	Vapor	Incapacitation
Mustard-T mixture	Vapor	Incapacitation
Lewisite	Vapor	Incapacitation
Mustard-lewisite mixture	Vapor	Incapacitation
Phenyldichloroarsine	Vapor	Incapacitation
Ethyldichloroarsine	Vapor	Incapacitation
Methyldichloroarsine	Vapor	Incapacitation
Phosgene oxime	Vapor	Coughing, choking, chest tightness on exposure; possible cyanosis following pulmonary edema

[a]NATO, 1996a; NRC, 1997a.
[b]Ali et al., 1997.
[c]Exposure via this route is unlikely; no information was found.

Sources: Boyle, 1998b; U.S. Army, 1995; U.S. Army et al., 1990.

Effective Dose (mg-min/m³ except where otherwise noted)	Rate of Action
$ICt_{50} = 7{,}000$	Very rapid
$ICt_{50} = 2{,}500$	Effects delayed from 2 hours to 11 days
$ICt_{50} = 150$ ECt_{50} = no existing estimates (threshold)[a] $ECt_{50} = 200$ (moderate temperature, severe effects)[a] $ECt_{50} = {>}50$ (mild effects)[a] $ECt_{50} = 10\text{–}1{,}000$[b]	Effects delayed for 4 to 6 hours
N/A[c]	Effects delayed for ~12 hours
N/A[c]	Delayed action not well known
$ECt_{50} = 1{,}500$	Rapid acting
N/A[c]	Rapid acting skin irritation, blisters in 13 hours
N/A[c]	Rapid acting
$ICt_{50} = 5\text{–}10$	Rapid acting nose/throat irritation, blisters in 12 hours
$ICt_{50} = 25$	Rapid acting nose/throat irritation, blisters in several hours
ICt_{50} = unknown; lowest irritant concentration after a 10 second exposure is 1 mg/m³; effects of the agent become unbearable after one minute at 3 mg/m³	Rapid acting

TABLE 2-6 Dermal Absorption Agents

Agent	Mode of Delivery	Effect
Tabun (GA)	Liquid; vapor	N/A[a]
Sarin (GB)	Liquid	N/A[a]
Soman (GD)	Liquid	N/A[a]
GF	Liquid	N/A[a]
VX	Liquid	N/A[a]
Distilled mustard	Liquid	Inflammation of the nose, throat, trachea, bronchi, and lungs
Nitrogen mustard	Liquid	Incapacitation
Mustard-T mixture	Liquid	Incapacitation
Lewisite	Liquid	Incapacitation
Mustard-lewisite mixture	Liquid	Incapacitation
Phenyldichloroarsine	Liquid	Incapacitation
Ethyldichloroarsine	Liquid	Incapacitation
Methyldichloroarsine	Liquid	Incapacitation

[a]Unlikely exposure via this route; no information found.
[b]Ali et al., 1997.
[c]NRC, 1997a.

Sources: Boyle, 1998b; NATO, 1996a; U.S. Army, 1995; U.S. Army et al., 1990.

Effective Dose (mg-min/m³ except where otherwise noted)	Rate of Action
ED_{50} = no existing estimates	Very rapid
ED_{50} = no existing estimates	Very rapid; may be lethal within 15 minutes of absorption
ED_{50} = no existing estimates	Very rapid; may be lethal within 15 minutes of absorption
ED_{50} = no existing estimates	Very rapid
ED_{50} = 5 mg/70-kg man[b] ED_{50} = 1 mg[c]	Very rapid; may be lethal within 15 minutes of absorption
ID_{50} = 2,000 by skin; 200 by eye ED_{50} = no existing estimates[b] ED_{50} = 10 Tg[c]	Effects delayed for 4 to 6 hours
ID_{50} = 200 by eye; 9,000 by skin	Effects delayed for ~12 hours
ID_{50} = very low	Delayed action not well known
ID_{50} = less than 300 by eye; more than 1,500 by skin ED_{50} = 15 Tg	Rapid acting
ID_{50} = 200 by eye; 1,500–2,000 by skin	Rapid acting skin irritation; blisters in 13 hours
ID_{50} = 16 as vomiting agent; 1,800 as blister	Rapid acting
N/A[a]	Rapid acting nose/throat irritation; blisters in 12 hours
N/A[a]	Rapid acting nose/throat irritation; blisters in several hours

TABLE 2-7 Dermal Necrotic Agents

Agent	Mode of Delivery	Effect
Distilled mustard	Liquid	Incapacitation
Nitrogen mustard	Liquid	Incapacitation
Mustard-T mixture	Liquid	Incapacitation
Mustard-lewisite mixture	Liquid	Incapacitation

[a] NATO, 1996a; NRC, 1997a.
[b] Ali et al., 1997.

Sources: Boyle, 1998b; U.S. Army, 1995; U.S. Army et al., 1990.

TABLE 2-8 Inhalation/Respiratory Agents

Agent	Mode of Delivery
Anthrax (*Bacillus anthracis*)	Aerosol
Plague (*Yersinia pestis*)	Aerosol
Tularemia (*Francisella tularensis*)	Aerosol
Q fever (*Coxiella burneti*)	Aerosol
Smallpox	Aerosol
Venezuelan equine encephalitis	Aerosol
Dysentery (*Shigella dysenteriae*)	Aerosol
Cholera (*Vibrio comma*)	Aerosol
Brucellolis (*Brucella suis*)	Aerosol

Sources: Ali et al., 1997; Boyle, 1998a; U.S. Air Force, 1997; U.S. Army et al., 1990.

Effective Dose	Rate of Action
$ID_{50} = 2{,}000$ by skin; 200 by eye ED_{50} = no existing estimates[a] $ED_{50} = 10$ μg[b]	Effects delayed for 4 to 6 hours
$ID_{50} = 200$ by eye; 9,000 by skin	Effects delayed for ~12 hours
ID_{50} = very low	Delayed action not well known
$ID_{50} = 200$ by eye; 1,500–2,000 by skin	Rapid acting skin irritation; blisters in 13 hours

Effect	Effective Dose	Onset Time (days)
75% morbidity; 80% mortality	8,000–50,000 spores	1–5
	100–500 organisms	2–3
80% morbidity; 35% mortality	10–50 organisms	2–3
70% morbidity; <1% mortality	1–10 organisms	14–21
30-35% mortality	10–100 organisms	12
90% morbidity; <5% mortality	10–100 organisms	1–5
25% mortality	10–100 organisms	1–7
15–90% mortality	1,000,000 organisms	1–5
2% fatality	10–100 organisms	5–21

TABLE 2-9 Ingestion Agents

Agent	Mode of Delivery
Anthrax (*Bacillus anthracis*)	Ingestion
Cholera (*Vibrio comma*)	Ingestion
Dysentery (*Shigella dysenteriae*)	Ingestion
Q Fever (*Coxiella burneti*)	Ingestion
Tularemia (*Francisella tularensis*)	Ingestion

[a]Information, if known, was not readily available during the course of the study.

Sources: Ali et al., 1997; Boyle, 1998a; U.S. Air Force, 1997; U.S. Army et al., 1990.

TABLE 2-10 Agents Absorbed via Mucous Membranes or the Skin

Agent	Mode of Delivery
Anthrax (*Bacillus anthracis*)	Direct contact with contaminated material
Tularemia (*Francisella tularensis*)	Inoculation of skin or mucous membranes with blood or tissue fluids of infected animals
Brucellosis (*Brucella suis*)	Through abraded and possibly intact skin
Ebola/Marburg	Through abrasion or via conjunctiva; possibly direct contact with blood or other tissues
Crimean-Congo hemorrhagic fever	Direct contact with animal or human tissues and blood

[a]Information, if known, was not readily available during the course of the study.

Sources: Ali et al., 1997; Boyle, 1998a; Johnson, 1990; LeDuc, 1989; Mikolich and Boyce, 1990; U.S. Air Force, 1997; U.S. Army et al., 1990.

THREAT AND RISK ASSESSMENT 51

Effect	Effective Dose	Onset Time (days)
75% morbidity; 80% mortality	1,000 spores	1–7
15–90% mortality	>10^7 organisms	1–5
25% mortality	10–100 organisms	1–7
70% morbidity; <1% mortality	1–10 organisms	14–21
80% morbidity; 35% mortality rate	N/A[a]	2–3

Effect	Effective Dose	Onset Time
25% mortality	N/A[a]	N/A[a]
80% morbidity; 35% mortality rate	10–50 organisms	N/A[a]
N/A[a]	N/A[a]	N/A[a]
N/A[a]	N/A[a]	N/A[a]
N/A[a]	N/A[a]	N/A[a]

Arthropod Vectors. Several threat agents can be carried by arthropods (e.g., flies, fleas, ticks, and mosquitoes). The agent is most often delivered by the insect's "bite," but other modes of contamination are possible. The number of agent organisms that represent an effective dose delivered by an arthropod and the effects and times of onset are shown in Table 2-11.

Threat Assessment

Threat assessments should be made for each type of conflict and every military operation. (See NRC report [1999c] for a framework for assessing risks to deployed forces in hostile environments.) Each level of military conflict or operation poses different challenges in terms of potential CB use and, therefore, different risks to deployed forces. Military operations range from major regional conflicts involving large numbers of personnel to policing and peacekeeping operations that involve small units. Therefore, commanders must have accurate, timely intelligence on the possible locations, quantities, and types of CB agents, as well as a knowledgeable CB advisor.

TABLE 2-11 Arthropod Vectors

Agent	Mode of Delivery
Plague (*Yersinia pestis*)	Fleas
Tularemia (*Francisella tularensis*)	Bites of infected deerflies, mosquitoes, or ticks
Rocky Mountain spotted fever (*Rickettsia rickettsi*)	Ticks
Yellow fever	Ticks
Rift Valley fever	Mosquitoes
Venezuelan equine encephalitis	Variety of mosquitoes
Crimean–Congo hemorrhagic fever	Ticks

[a]Information, if known, was not readily available during the course of the study.
Sources: Ali et al., 1997; Boyle, 1998a; LeDuc, 1989; U.S. Air Force, 1997; U.S. Army et al., 1990.

RISK MINIMIZATION/PROTECTION OF PERSONNEL

The most obvious way to minimize risk from exposure to CB agents is to avoid contact with these materials. The military has developed a four-part strategy for protecting deployed forces based on avoiding exposure: sensing, shaping, shielding, and sustaining. Sensing the NBC conditions throughout the joint battle space is accomplished by means of surveillance, detection, identification, monitoring, and reconnaissance. Shaping includes situation awareness of the battle space and managing, assessing, and recording threats (see the Task 2.2 report [NRC, 1999b]). Shielding joint and coalition forces includes medical pretreatment, personal protective equipment (PPE) and collective protective equipment (CPE). Sustaining the force after NBC attacks includes medical treatment and decontamination.

Avoiding contact depends on the capability and availability of detection equipment. Because the lag in detection time of our present capabilities (10 to 15 minutes) is longer than the time it takes to don protective equipment (Table 2-12), (NRC, 1999b), our current capability has been

Effect	Effective Dose	Onset Time (days)
25–100% mortality	$1-10^3$ organisms	2–7
80% morbidity; 35% mortality	$1-10^3$ organisms	1–10
7–20% fatal	N/A^a	3–10
< 5% mortality	N/A^a	3–6
< 1% mortality	N/A^a	3–12
90% morbidity; <5% mortality	$1-10^3$ organisms	4–20
N/A^a	N/A^a	N/A^a

TABLE 2-12 Time to Achieve MOPP 4

	MOPP LEVELS				
	MOPP0	MOPP 1	MOPP 2	MOPP 3	MOPP 4
Overgarment	Available	Worn	Worn	Worn	Worn
Boots	Available	Available	Worn	Worn	Worn
Mask	Carried	Carried	Carried	Worn	Worn
Gloves	Carried	Carried	Carried	Carried	Worn
Time to MOPP 4 (min)	8	4	0.5	0.25	0

called "detect to treat" (Cain, 1999). A preventive, rather than responsive, posture would be advantageous, of course, but this will require better detection capability.

In 1998, seven joint CB future operational capabilities (FOCs) (i.e., operational capabilities required to develop warfighting concepts to guide military and industrial R&D) were identified (Payne, 1998). One FOC focuses on the need for detecting and identifying prelaunch indicators, launch signatures, flight paths, and release or impact point(s) of theater missiles, including the ability to distinguish between conventional and NBC munitions. The detection system must provide early and selective warning and must be compatible with the current and future joint command, control, communications, computer, and intelligence (C4I) structure; warning and reporting systems; and NBC battle management systems. Because the FOC is far beyond present detection technologies, personnel must be protected by the combined use of PPE, CPE, and medical protective services.

The military approach to individual protection is embodied in the concept called Mission Oriented Protective Posture (MOPP), an ensemble of protective garments, boots, masks, and gloves. MOPP-Ready status is defined as having protective garments available; MOPP 4 status is defined as all components of the protective ensemble being worn. The progression is shown in Table 2-13.

CB battlefield exigencies may require collective protection, a place for medical treatment of casualties and the removal of MOPP gear for eating and recovery periods. Therefore, protective shelters have been developed based on filtering and overpressurization technologies. If individuals or

TABLE 2-13 Levels of Mission-Oriented Protective Posture (MOPP)

MOPP Ready	Soldiers carry protective masks with their load-carrying equipment. The soldier's MOPP gear is labeled and stored no further back than the battalion support area and is ready to be brought forward to the soldier when needed. The time necessary to bring the MOPP gear forward will not exceed two hours. A second set of MOPP gear is available within six hours. Units at MOPP-Ready are highly vulnerable to attacks with persistent agents and will automatically upgrade to MOPP-Zero when they determine, or are notified, that chemical weapons have been used or that the threat of chemical weapons has arisen. When a unit is at MOPP-Ready, soldiers will have field-expedient items identified for use.
MOPP 0	Soldiers carry protective masks with their load-carrying equipment. The standard battledress overgarment and other individual protective equipment that make up the soldier's MOPP gear are readily available (i.e., equipment is either carried by each soldier or stored within arm's reach [e.g., within the work area, vehicle, or fighting position]). Units at MOPP Zero are highly vulnerable to attacks with persistent agents and will automatically upgrade to MOPP 1 when they determine, or are notified, that persistent chemical weapons have been used or that the threat of chemical weapons has arisen.
MOPP 1	When directed to MOPP 1, soldiers immediately don battledress overgarments. In hot weather, the overgarment jacket may be unbuttoned and the battledress overgarment may be worn directly over the underwear. M9 or M8 chemical detection paper is attached to the overgarment. MOPP 1 provides a great deal of protection against persistent agents. The level is automatically assumed when chemical weapons have been used in an area of operations or when directed by higher command.
MOPP 2	Soldiers put on chemical protective footwear covers, green vinyl overboots, or a field-expedient item (e.g., vapor-barrier boots), and the protective helmet cover. The overgarment jacket may be left unbuttoned, but the trousers remain closed.
MOPP 3	Soldiers wear protective masks and hoods. Flexibility is built into the system to allow the soldier relief at MOPP 3. Particularly in hot weather, soldiers may open the overgarment jacket and roll the protective mask hood for ventilation, but the trousers remain closed.

TABLE 2-13 Levels of Mission-Oriented Protective Posture (MOPP) (continued)

MOPP 4	Soldiers will completely encapsulate themselves by closing their overgarments, rolling down and adjusting mask floods, and putting on the NBC rubber gloves with cotton liners. MOPP 4 provides the highest degree of chemical protection, but it also has the most negative impact on performance.
Mask Only	Only the protective mask is worn. The mask-only command is given in these situations: (1) when riot control agents are being employed and no chemical or biological threat exists; and (2) in a downwind vapor hazard of a nonpersistent chemical agent. The Mask-Only command is not appropriate when blister agents or persistent nerve agents are present.

Source: U.S. Army Office of the Surgeon General, 1997.

equipment are contaminated, however, they must be decontaminated prior to entry into a collective protection area.

Medical treatments can afford additional protection both before and after exposure (IOM, 1999a). Individual protection, collective protection, and decontamination are three means of risk minimization, and each has an associated doctrinal, training, and R&D component.

FINDINGS AND RECOMMENDATION

The following findings are based on information provided for this study during briefings and discussions with individuals involved with the CB RDA process.

Finding. Joint structure and joint service processes were developed to maximize the efficient use of funds and to reduce duplications of effort.

Finding. The purpose of the joint prioritization of system needs (and, therefore, RDA needs) is to ensure that fielded systems meet joint service needs. This requires that CINC priorities and NBC community priorities be coordinated.

Finding. The prioritization and selection of RDA projects are often based on compromises or political trade-offs unrelated to CINC prioritization, technical capabilities, or *bona fide* needs and are focused on service-specific, rather than joint service, needs.

Finding. System development is sometimes based on outdated and possibly inaccurate evaluations of threats and challenges.

Recommendation. The Department of Defense should reevaluate and possibly revise its prioritization process for the development of equipment. The reevaluation should include a reassessment of the use of threat information.

3

Philosophy, Doctrine, and Training for Chemical and Biological Warfare

PHILOSOPHY

DoD has an active CB defense program as well as a passive defense program (DoD, 1996). The active program involves improving capabilities for detecting, tracking, identifying, intercepting, destroying, and neutralizing NBC warheads delivered by airborne launch platforms, ballistic missiles, and cruise missiles, while minimizing collateral effects. The passive defense program involves protecting against the effects of CB weapons. The passive defense programs includes: (1) contamination avoidance (reconnaissance, detection, and warning); (2) force protection (individual protection, collective protection, and medical support); and (3) decontamination.

Contamination avoidance includes sensors for joint task forces, mobile CB reconnaissance, and systems capable of detecting multiple CB agents and characterizing new agents. Technological advances to support this policy include remote detectors, miniaturization, lower detection limits, logistics support, and biological detection capability.

In force protection, improved mask systems and advanced protective clothing are being developed under a joint program to reduce the weight, heat stress, and logistics burden of current gear. (See Chapter 4 for a description.) Medical research is directed toward improving prophylaxes, antidotes, treatments, vaccines, and medical casualty management. Other research is focused on lightweight CB protective shelters and collective protection technologies (see Chapter 4).

In decontamination, modular systems are being developed, and new

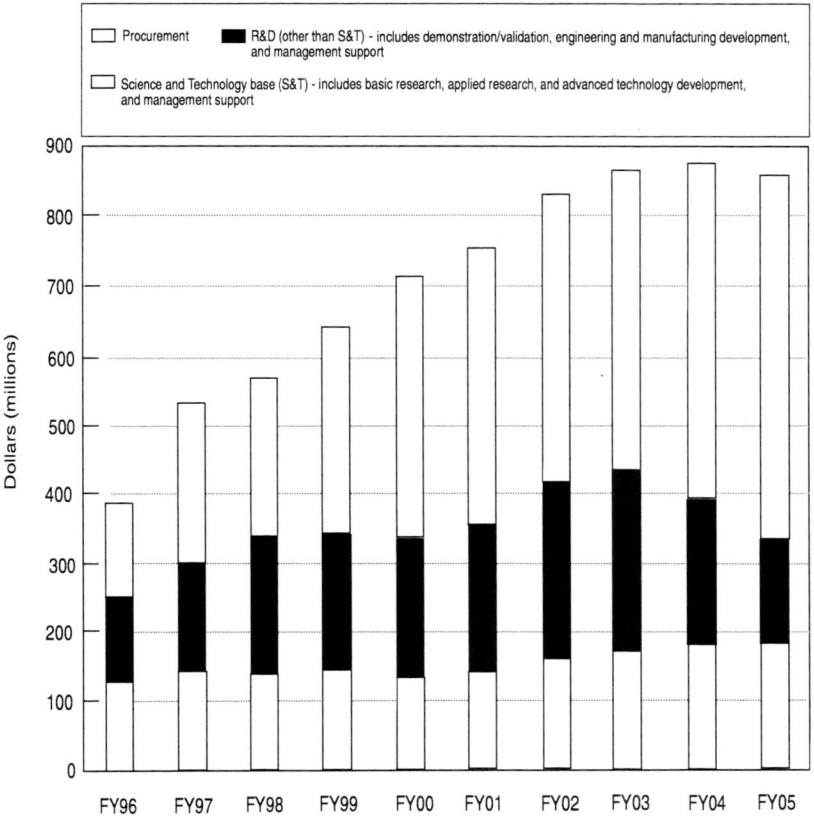

FIGURE 3-1 Summary of appropriations for the Chemical and Biological Defense Program.

technologies, such as sorbents, catalytic coatings, and the physical removal of contaminants, are being developed (DoD, 1996).

RDT&E and procurement budgets for the joint service CB defense program have steadily increased from about $388 million in fiscal year (FY) 1996 to the current level of $645 million in FY 1999 (DoD, 1999). Figure 3-1 provides a summary of appropriated and requested funding from FY 1996 to FY 2005. As the funding profiles show, funding levels for the science and technology base (i.e., basic research, applied research, and advanced technology development) are relatively stable. Based on these figures and the funds for individual protection, collective protection, and decontamination technologies (see Appendix A for a detailed breakout of the funds), new technologies for physical protection and decontamination are not likely to be developed.

DoD established an integrated CB defense program under the oversight of the Deputy Assistant to the Secretary of Defense for Counter-Proliferation and Chemical/Biological Defense (DATSD [CP/CBD]). This program was created to consolidate, coordinate, and integrate the CB defense requirements of all services into a single program. DoD also established the Counterproliferation Support Program specifically to address shortfalls in operational capabilities. The Counterproliferation Support Program supports the following existing programs to accelerate the deployment of essential military counterproliferation technologies and capabilities: (1) a program to accelerate (by up to six years) the fielding of an advanced, long-range, eye-safe, infrared LIDAR (laser detection device) to provide long-range battlefield warning of CB agents; (2) a program to evaluate the use of ultraviolet multifrequency lasers to detect and characterize biological agents by their fluorescent spectra; (3) a program to develop miniaturized CB extremely sensitive point detectors that can be installed on unmanned aerial vehicles; (4) a program to accelerate (by two years) the procurement of improved PPE and CPE; (5) a program to expand the technology base for decontamination; and (6) a program to improve joint NBC doctrine and training procedures by improving battlefield simulations (DoD, 1996). Approximately $30 million was budgeted in FY 1996 to support these programs. In addition, the Counterproliferation Support Program supports the activities of the CB defense program and facilitates the collection of information on proliferant states.

The Defense Threat Reduction Agency carries out the CB technology development activities (referred to as the "tech base") for the DATSD (CP/CBD) through the Joint Technology Panel for Chemical and Biological Defense. The CB tech base includes programs for the development of active defenses and a number of passive defenses. The Army's programs also include the operation of Dugway Proving Ground, Utah, as the primary test range for CB defensive equipment. Details on CB testing at Dugway can be found in reports by the Counterproliferation Program Review Committee issued in May 1995 and 1997 (DoD, 1995, 1997a).

CHEMICAL/BIOLOGICAL WARFARE DOCTRINE

Past Doctrine: "Fight Dirty"

Before systems for detecting contaminated areas were available, military planners developed a doctrine (best described as the "fight dirty" doctrine) that supported operations in contaminated areas. The doctrine involved a combination of individual protective equipment and extensive training to enable individuals and units to fight in contaminated environments. Individual protective equipment (MOPP) consisted of heavy carbon-impregnated materials, ill-fitting restrictive masks, and heavy protective gloves and boots. The protective masks required special filters to absorb airborne agents and protect the lungs and eyes. The other components protected against agent contact with the skin—in solid, liquid, or vapor form. Impermeable overboots and butyl rubber gloves provided a solid barrier to liquid agents. Overgarments and hoods were designed to permit some passage of air and moisture, allowing perspiration to evaporate, but they were impractical for most combat functions because the rapid buildup of body heat and moisture quickly rendered soldiers nonfunctional. Garments were designed with two layers, an outer layer that limited liquid absorption or redistributed it to reduce concentration and an inner layer (constructed of charcoal-impregnated foam) that filtered the air and adsorbed any vapor that penetrated the outer layer.

Because detection and warning systems were (and still are) inadequate (see NRC, 1999b), MOPP 4 has been consistently overused in training exercises (Williams, 1998). Anecdotal reports indicate that the same was true in Desert Shield/Desert Storm (NRC, 1999d), which resulted in significant decrements in unit effectiveness because of heat load, restricted vision, and loss of tactile sensitivity.

Current Doctrine: Contamination Avoidance

As technologies have advanced, especially detection technologies, and as new, more capable detection equipment has been fielded (e.g., the automatic chemical agent detection alarm), the doctrine has shifted to "contamination avoidance." The basis of this doctrine is that U.S. forces can now engage an enemy while avoiding casualties from contamination by CB agents. Avoiding contamination requires rapid and accurate detection, identification, warning, and reporting systems for the presence of threat agents. Protective equipment and decontamination systems are still necessary, however, in situations where avoidance of contamination is impossible (e.g., fixed sites) or for missions that require operations in a contaminated environment.

CHEMICAL/BIOLOGICAL WARFARE TRAINING

Once the new doctrine of contamination avoidance (with concomitant detection and chemical protective equipment) was adopted, training was naturally modified to implement it. A critical requirement for deterring the use of CB agents (and for successful operations if deterrence fails) is that forces be fully trained to respond to the full spectrum of CB threats. At the most basic level, CB training includes learning how to don boots, gloves, masks, and overgarments and how to conduct battlefield operations in a CB environment using protective equipment. Training requires repetition and commitment on the part of unit commanders and is relatively straightforward in execution. Discussions (at Fort Benning and at NRC workshop) with individual soldiers who have undergone this training in the last several years revealed that the commitment to CB training is left to the unit commander's discretion and that training has been inconsistent, both within and across services. Thus, some equipment shortfalls may have been exacerbated by inadequate training and could be mitigated by more consistent and more stringent training (including training with coalition forces).

Although shortcomings in the training of individuals can be easily overcome, training commanders at all levels to react to a potential CB environment is quite difficult. Commanders must be taught to determine when protective gear is necessary, what levels of protection are necessary, and the timing and methods of removing MOPP gear safely. An audit conducted by the DoD Office of the Inspector General assessing unit training in chemical and biological defense revealed that commanders were not fully integrating CB defense into their unit training (DoD, 1998a). As a result, "commanders could not adequately assess unit readiness to successfully complete wartime missions under chemical and biological conditions" (DoD, 1998a, p.1). Both commanders and individual soldiers must have a realistic idea of the risk in a given situation (see section "Understanding the Risk" below).

The current state of CB training has been reviewed in numerous documents (e.g., DoD, 1998a, 1999; Joseph, 1996), and DoD has acknowledged that the integration of safe, realistic CB defense, including defense against aerosol agents, into training simulations is essential. Models and simulations could be used to enable both units and commanders to understand an adversary's intent and CB capabilities and to enable trainees to visualize how CB capabilities might affect the battle space, defensive responses, and planned operations. Models and simulations would also enable commanders to apply CB defense training doctrine and leader-development training strategies in preparing their forces to maintain operational continuity and fulfill their missions in a CB environment. Currently, several engineering-level models represent the dynamics of CB contamination, but only a few robust representations of chemical effects (and almost none for biological effects) have been fully implemented in war games; and few analytical models have been used for training (DoD, 1999; Joseph, 1996).

> There is inadequate guidance within the services or from operational chains of command that defines tasks, conditions, or standards for more complex CBW activities such as operational planning to minimize the potential effects of enemy NBC use...the commanders of units

undergoing training essentially determine the scope and nature of play, if any, to be included in the scenarios by CTC [Combat Training Center] controllers and opposing forces (Joseph, 1996, p. 78).

UNDERSTANDING THE RISK

Commanders are much better able to assess the hazards posed by the familiar risks from ballistic weapons than from CB weapons. The lack of information concerning how CB agents affect health and at what concentrations they are dangerous has skewed the overall perception of risk and has led to DoD adopting the goal of complete CB protection with no, or minimal, casualties. Thus, the level of protection from CB threats is higher (100 percent) than the level of protection from ballistic threats.

The 100-percent protection level has resulted in overly conservative choices for protection against unrealistically high challenge levels. Protective equipment has been designed to meet CB challenges that are far greater than realistic battlefield threats. For example, many countries believed to possess CB capabilities may not have suitable delivery systems to create a sustainable threat of the magnitude against which the United States is currently defending (see Table 3-1 for service-specific requirements for liquid and vapor contamination levels) (Institute for Defense Analyses, 1999).

Even though some enemies could contaminate a given target to this level, the requirement for percutaneous protection should not be determined on this basis. The requirement should balance inherent risk factors and trade-offs between the protection of the individual and the combat effectiveness of the force. The implicit assumption of maximum CB protection is that it will minimize casualties. In fact, the opposite may be true because a protective system that significantly encumbers the soldier will degrade the overall combat effectiveness of the unit (see Chapter 4). This

TABLE 3-1 Service Requirements for JSLIST

Challenge Levels	Army	Navy-Sea	Air Force-Ground	Marines
Liquid protection (g/m^2)	10	5	5	10
Vapor protection ($mg*min/m^3$)	$10,000^a/5,000^b$	5,000	7,500	no standard

[a]For Army aviators and all CB undergarments
[b]Overgarment

Source: Barrett, 1998.

degradation affects all units that don protective gear, regardless of whether or not their location has actually been targeted. The decrease in combat effectiveness across the larger force may result in more overall casualties than may have resulted from a lesser protective posture with less of an effect on combat performance.

Contamination is not usually uniform in a target area. Contamination levels are likely to be significantly higher than the challenge against which the United States currently defends in some areas but significantly lower elsewhere. In fact, the areas with the highest contamination densities will be closest to the burst of the munitions. Consequently, ballistic fragmentation effects are also likely to be highest in these same areas. Some analyses have suggested that the ballistics effects of bursting chemical multiple launch rocket system (MLRS) rounds may have as much as 30 percent of the ballistics effects of a comparable high-explosive MLRS round (Battelle Memorial Institute and Charles Williams, Inc., 1999). This means that significant portions of those areas with 10 g/m^2 or greater liquid agent contamination densities would also be subject to lethal shell-fragment effects (Institute for Defense Analyses, 1999). Thus, chemical protective suits would be ineffective in these areas, regardless of the level of contamination.

Striking a balance between protection and performance will require that many factors be considered. Specifically, the intelligence community must assess the enemy's overall ability to deliver a CB agent on target. Planners need to know how many and what types of targets might be contaminated to the level against which the United States currently protects (Table 3-1), the delivery systems that might be used, and the enemy's resupply capabilities before the appropriate assessments can be made. As the number of U.S. forces and resources continue to decline, U.S. intelligence will have to provide these types of assessments so that the current totally risk-averse position can be adjusted to a realistic risk management strategy.

Current appraisals of the threat and current toxicological information are inadequate for proper evaluations of the health consequences of exposure, even with soldiers in MOPP 4 status. Evaluations of the protection afforded by various MOPP levels are based on estimates of the CB dose that can be delivered to an individual. Although some simulant studies have been conducted, they may not be universally applicable to all CB agents, especially aerosol agents (NRC, 1997b). The existing toxicological data on real agents are sparse. In recent reports, previous studies on the toxicity of chemical agents in humans and animals have been reevaluated to determine reference doses (NRC, 1997a, 1999e). However, these data are not reliable enough for the purposes of modeling and simulation for the following reasons: (1) not enough data have been collected; (2) the assays used to collect these data are not as sensitive as advanced methods; and (3) they do not show subtle effects. Therefore, modelers have determined that they do not have sufficient information on toxicokinetic factors, such as the uptake, metabolism, and excretion of CB agents, to predict risks and hazards accurately. These circumstances have led to an exaggerated perception of risk and a design for overprotection.

According to information presented at briefings and in a previous NRC report (e.g., Institute for Defense Analyses, 1999; NRC, 1985; U.S. Army SBCCOM, 1998), little evidence supports the hypothesis that low-level exposures to CB agents have long-term deleterious health effects. However, because of a lack of data, substantial doubts have been raised, and illnesses that cannot be medically diagnosed or attributed to conventional causes may be attributed to CB exposures (NRC, 1999b). Since FY 1996, DoD has dedicated $5 million to evaluating the chronic effects of low-level exposures to chemical agents (DoD, 1999). Studies have been under way since the first quarter of 1997 to develop highly specific and sensitive assay equipment that can be used in forward areas to detect and potentially quantify low-level exposures to chemical agents. According to the Executive Summary of the Persian Gulf Veterans Coordinating Board Action Plan with Respect to the Findings and Recommendations of the Presidential Advisory Committee (1997, p. 2),

> Federal research requests for proposals include the possible long-term health effects of chemical and other hazards (including subclinical exposure to CW [chemical warfare] nerve agents)...[and there is] development of a strategic plan for research into the potential health consequences of exposure to chemical or other hazards, including low levels of chemical agents.

In May 1999, the U.S. Army Center for Health Promotion and Preventive Medicine published Technical Guide (TG) 230A, *Short Term Chemical Exposure Guidelines for Deployed Military Personnel*, to address the health risks that may be experienced by deployed military personnel following temporary or short-term exposure to a number of toxic chemicals (U.S. Army CHPPM, 1999). These guidelines are based on a variety of effects, ranging from mild signs or symptoms and long-term delayed effects from low-level exposures, to more severe effects, such as death, from temporary high-level exposures. Commanders must be trained and evaluated on the appropriate use of these new guidelines. A second technical guidance document (TG 230B), which will address the risks associated with longer-term exposures (i.e., from 14 days to one year), is under development.

FINDINGS AND RECOMMENDATIONS

Finding. The battlefield areas with the highest contamination levels will also have the highest levels of ballistic fragmentation lethalities. Therefore, CB protective measures will be ineffective in these areas regardless of the liquid or vapor challenge levels. The threat from CB weapons relative to other battlefield threats is unknown.

Recommendation. The Department of Defense should reevaluate liquid and vapor challenge levels based on the most current threat information and use the results in the materiel requirements process and, subsequently, in the development of training programs and doctrine.

Finding. Little or no new funding is being provided for basic research on new technologies for physical protection and decontamination.

Recommendation. The Department of Defense should reprogram funds to alleviate the shortfall in basic research on new technologies for physical protection and decontamination.

Finding. Unit commanders receive little training related to assessing CB risks to their units, especially in determinating when, whether, and how much protective gear is necessary.

Recommendation. The Department of Defense should develop commander training protocols and/or simulations to assist unit leaders in making appropriate chemical and biological risk-based decisions.

4

Physical Protection

Traditional individual and collective protective techniques represent one way to avoid injury from chemical or biological weapons. An alternative approach would be to move the individual or unit out of harm's way. This approach might involve seeding clouds to cause rainfall to remove CB agents, generating wind to "blow" agents away from troops, or spreading troops out to decrease the likelihood that large numbers will be contaminated. These nontraditional techniques may be appropriate subjects for future studies but are beyond the scope of this study.

INDIVIDUAL PROTECTION

Risks and Challenges

The need to protect individuals in a CB environment was prompted by (1) respiratory and mucous membrane threats, which led to the development of masks and filters, and (2) the advent of chemical agents that attacked via the skin (percutaneously) as well as via the respiratory system, which led to the development of personal protective garments and other physical barriers. Currently, PPE consists of a mask, special overgarments, and gloves and boots. Used collectively or in various combinations, the equipment is called MOPP. Army *FM 3-4* defines various combinations of MOPP gear in terms of protection levels, depending on perceived battlefield conditions.

In an ideal situation, protective equipment could be donned in the field without encumbering the wearer. Unfortunately, state-of-the art gear is cumbersome, creates severe thermal stress, and interferes with the effective use of weapons systems. In addition, some individuals have had adverse physical reactions to the materials used in the construction of protective equipment and adverse psychological reactions to its use. To mitigate these difficulties, the Army has developed a strategy that combines doctrine, training, and equipment to enable U.S. forces to operate as effectively as possible in a CB environment.

Current Doctrine and Training

Mission-Oriented Protective Posture (MOPP)

Originally, there were five MOPP levels, ranging from MOPP 0 to MOPP 4, the highest level of protection in which all gear must be worn. In 1996, Change 2 to *FM 3-4* increased the number of MOPP levels from five to seven, as shown in Table 2-13 (U.S. Army and U.S. Marine Corps, 1992). The two new MOPP levels are MOPP Ready and Mask Only. The Mask Only level is used either when riot control agents are used and there is no CB threat, when forces are downwind of a nonpersistent chemical agent, or when a biological threat is believed to be nonpercutaneous. However, MOPP levels are not fixed or rigid. Commanders are responsible for determining the protective posture of their subordinate units and for deciding whether to modify a MOPP level. The effectiveness of MOPP training is limited by the constraints imposed by the equipment. For example, it may be impossible to go from a Mask-Only status to MOPP 4 without temporarily breaching the mask seal. To make best use of MOPP equipment, even with its drawbacks, will require effective training.

Protection of U.S. forces from the effects of CB agents must be based on an understanding of their effects, which depend on the characteristics and properties of these agents. Obviously, the most important factor is the nature of the agent, including its toxicity, its mechanism of action, its mode of entry into the victim, and its persistence in the environment. However, other factors, such as meteorological conditions, are also critical. Wind speed, wind direction, atmospheric stability (e.g., inversions), temperature, humidity, and intensity of sunlight can limit or enhance the effectiveness of the initial attack and influence the persistence and concentration of the agent in the target area.

Lethal and incapacitating doses for selected chemical agents are shown in Table 4-1. "Liquid hazard" refers to the level of liquid film that constitutes a significant hazard (10 percent of lethal dose) to unprotected personnel. Vapor challenges can occur when individuals are exposed to the initial vapor cloud and as vapor is generated by the evaporation of liquid films on contaminated surfaces. Vapor challenges are shown in

TABLE 4-1 Approximate Toxicity of Chemical Agents

	Route of Exposure	Liquid Hazard (mg/m^2)	Vapor Challenge (mg-min/m^3)		
			LCT_{50}	ICT_{50}	$OCT_{threshold}$
Choking Agents					
Phosgene (CG)	respiratory		3,200	1,600	
Blistering Agents					
Mustard (HD)	respiratory		900	450	60
	percutaneous	~700	1,500	750	
Blood Agents					
Hydrogen cyanide (AC)			2,000–4,500	varies	
Nerve Agents					
Tabun (GA)	respiratory		270	200	
	percutaneous	~50	30,000	15,000	2.5
Sarin (GB)	respiratory		35	20	
	percutaneous	~170	10,000	5,000	1.5
Soman (GD)	respiratory		70	35	
	percutaneous	~15	10,000	5,000	0.2
VX	respiratory		15	8	
	percutaneous	~0.5	150	75	0.06

Note: Percutaneous values are for bare skin.

Source: U.S. Army Chemical Defense Equipment Process Action Team, 1994.

units of concentration × time (mg-min/m^3). For example, incapacitation is assumed to be possible if an unprotected individual is exposed by inhalation to tabun (GA) at 200 mg/m^3 for 1 minute or to 20 mg/m^3 for 10 minutes.

With sufficient warning time and accessibile PPE, effective protection can be achieved. The protective gear currently in development promises significant improvements over previous models. The new mask (the joint service general purpose mask [JSGPM]) will allow for better peripheral vision, should be more comfortable to wear, and will have a somewhat flexible design to meet specific service requirements (e.g., allowing Air Force personnel to perform a Valsalva maneuver to equalize pressure in their ears). A joint service lightweight integrated suit (JSLIST), which has been developed and is being fielded, is an overgarment that can be worn in place of the regular uniform. The JSLIST is constructed of a single-layer material that allows for the transport of water through the material but traps or repels CB agents. The materials used in the construction of the gloves and boots, however, have not changed.

The previous MOPP gear had serious drawbacks, the most important of which was interference with performance at the MOPP 4 level (DoD, 1997b). To minimize the thermal stresses imposed by the vapor-impervious battledress overgarment (BDO), individuals were forced to greatly reduce their level of effort. The work-rest cycle, according to requirements documents, was 16 minutes of work followed by about 44 minutes of rest in each hour. According to specifications, the new JSLIST garment allows individuals to work for 43 minutes and rest for 17 minutes, which is a dramatic improvement in efficiency. The Joint Operational Requirements Document for the JSLIST states that the JSLIST overgarment requirements be met when the warfighter is engaged in moderate activity (450 Watts), at 32.2°C with 50 percent relative humidity, and a three to five mile-per-hour wind (U.S. Marine Corps, 1999a). In most situations, however, individuals do not wear the protective clothing throughout a deployment, and they must be able to don protective gear quickly and efficiently. Therefore, the most important link in the protection chain is the early detection and warning of an attack.

Studies of the time it takes personnel to advance to MOPP 4 were conducted at the U.S. Army Chemical School in 1992. The results are summarized in Table 4-2.[1] If personnel have sufficient warning time to reach MOPP 4 level, casualties will be minimal. To reach MOPP 4 posture at least eight minutes of warning time is required for an individual wearing no MOPP gear at all. Most currently fielded warning and detection systems cannot provide that much advance notice. In addition, some CB attack scenarios allow no time for response. For example, in the event of an attack by tactical ballistic missiles, the attack and launch early reporting to theater (ALERT) system, which was activated in 1995, can provide three to four minutes advance warning. Thus, troops at MOPP 0 directly below a burst would be exposed to chemical agents for up to eight minutes. If the agent were GD and vapor concentrations were 7 mg/m^3 for five minutes (equal to 35 mg-min/m^3 or LCt_{50}), casualties could be extremely heavy (Institute for Defense Analyses, 1999). In general, the distance of troops from the center of a CB attack will determine whether they have adequate time to don MOPP gear.

---

[1]Table 4-2 includes a category of protective posture, MOPP 0.5, that is not included in current doctrine. MOPP 0.5 is a protective posture recently introduced by the Air Force, at which the mask, gloves, and boots, but not the overgarment, are worn. This protective posture, which has not been adopted by the joint services, has been found to be effective for operations at a "transfer base" (Chow et al., 1998).

TABLE 4-2 Time to Achieve MOPP 4

	MOPP LEVELS					
	MOPP 0	USAF MOPP 0.5	MOPP 1	MOPP 2	MOPP 3	MOPP 4
Overgarment	Available	Available	Worn	Worn	Worn	Worn
Boots	Available	Worn	Available	Worn	Worn	Worn
Mask	Carried	Worn	Carried	Carried	Worn	Worn
Gloves	Carried	Worn	Carried	Carried	Carried	Worn
Time to MOPP 4 (min)	8	~8	4	0.5	0.25	0

Source: Chow et al., 1998.

Effective Training

Even with the old PPE, the level of protection could be increased and deficiencies reduced (although not eliminated) with proper training. Conversely, regardless of the quality of the equipment, inadequate training leads to improper use and inefficient or inadequate protection. Discussions with individuals who have served in units trained for operations in CB environments indicated that the quality and intensity of training both within and across services is inconsistent, reflecting the different priorities assigned to CB training by individual commanders (Committee on Veterans' Affairs, 1998; DoD, 1998a).

Relating Risk to Doctrine/Equipment

The risk of exposure to most CB agents are, in decreasing order, inhalation, ocular penetration, and percutaneous penetration. The order for donning protective equipment, therefore, should be mask, gloves, overgarment, and boots. Because of limitations in equipment design, however, it may not be possible to don equipment in this order. No data were found during this study to indicate that this issue has been adequately investigated.

Design criteria for PPE include withstanding challenges of 10 g/m^2 for liquid contaminants and vapor challenges of 5,000 to 10,000 $mg\text{-}min/m^3$. Modeling data have confirmed that these contamination levels may be attained in limited areas for short periods of time. However, no intelligence studies have shown that any current potential adversary could mount a battlefield attack that would attain these levels for an extended period of time or across an extended geographical area (Institute for Defense Analyses, 1999). If the requirement of protecting against this threat level were relaxed, PPE that would be more supportive of the individual soldier and less detrimental to unit effectiveness could be developed.

The underlying philosophy of the CB R&D defense programs is based on the doctrine of contamination avoidance. R&D on PPE supports the doctrine by developing equipment that provides protection while reducing negative impacts on mission-related activities. Major efforts have been devoted to the development of the fibers, cloths, and adsorbents used in the construction of PPE. R&D in these areas is briefly described in the next section (for more details see Appendix B).

In spite of the protective clothing and equipment used by deployed forces, casualties will still occur from CB agents, ballistic fragmentation, or some other source. The effective and efficient management of casualties in a contaminated environment will require that procedures be in place for first aid, other medical treatment, evacuation, and decontamination. Current U.S. Army Medical Department doctrine emphasizes the treatment of casualties as far forward as possible and the timely and efficient evacuation of casualties.

Task 2.4 of the overall deployed forces study addresses the medical treatment of casualty management (IOM, 1999a). However, protocols and equipment for patient protection, transporting casualties, and decontaminating casualties are also necessary. Current doctrine addresses these issues only on a general level, leaving much of the decision making to unit commanders. The doctrine for casualty management can be found in various places, including: (1) Joint Publication 4-02, Doctrine for Health Service Support in Joint Operations, which describes the requirements for health service support in an NBC environment; (2) NATO Handbook on the Medical Aspects of NBC Defensive Operations (NATO, 1996a, 1996b); (3) the Treatment of Chemical Casualties and Conventional Military Chemical Injuries (*FM 8-285*) (U.S. Army et al., 1995); (4) Medical Evacuation in Specific Environments (*FM 8-10-6*) (U.S. Army, 1991a); (5) Health Service Support in an NBC Environment (*FM 8-10-7*) (U.S. Army, 1993); and (6) NBC Decontamination (*FM 3-5*) (U.S. Army and U.S. Marine Corps, 1993).

Casualties serious enough to warrant evacuation are transported by three basic modes: personnel, ground vehicles, and aircraft (aircraft are the least available transport vehicles). According to doctrine, once a vehicle is contaminated, it is restricted to working in "dirty" environments so they do not have to be decontaminated while they are needed in operations and they do not contaminate clean environments.

Textiles and Garments

Textiles and garments are the "second skins" of a soldier, the barriers between soldiers and the surrounding environment. Although the global and national political climate has changed, and defense concepts and doctrines with them, the basic role of clothing in protecting the soldier has remained the same. In the increasingly complex battlefield environment, the fundamental question is whether textile and garment manufacturing technologies are keeping pace with current and future demands.

This section reviews the requirements for CB protection, current barrier concepts, current material systems, and the fabric engineering approach for improving the protective capability of textiles and garments. These descriptions are followed by an assessment of the current state of readiness of the U.S. fiber-textile-garment industry to meet the needs of future soldiers and an identification of the key issues that remain to be addressed in the development of chemical protective textiles and garments.

TABLE 4-3 Requirements for Chemical Protective Textiles

- Reduced heat stress
- Reduced weight-to-bulk ratio
- Skin compatibility
- Combat uniform configuration
- Longer service life
- Longer shelf life
- Fire resistance
- Easier laundering
- Capability of being decontaminated
- Reusability
- Durability
- Camouflage capability
- Water repellency
- Resistance to perspiration
- Resistance to petroleum products
- Nontoxicity of materials
- Compatibility with other items

Source: Roth, 1982.

The technical requirements for CB protective textiles are summarized in Table 4-3. These requirements can be evaluated in terms of four key properties: weight, bulk, durability (wear time-protection time), and comfort (which includes ease of vision, breathing, and movement, as well as heat stress).

Clothing

R&D to improve PPE has led to the development of some long-term goals (shown schematically in Table 4-4). As an example of the evolution of fabrics, the technologies used for the OG84/BDO (the ®Saratoga chemical protective overgarment), and the JSLIST are compared in Table 4-4.

Modifications in textile materials, including fibers, yarn, and fabric structures, can reduce weight and bulk, improve durability, and reduce heat stress. To reduce weight, fibers of lower density and yarn and fabric structures with low packing density can be used. Smaller fiber diameters and higher packing density can reduce bulkiness. Smaller fiber diameters can be achieved using an electrospinning process, in which a polymer solution is exposed to an electrical field that elongates the polymer jet to form fibers ranging from 50 to 150 nm in diameter (Reneker and Chun, 1996). This process has been demonstrated successfully for a wide range of polymers at the Fibrous Materials Research Center at Drexel University and at several government laboratories (Gibson et al., 1999; Ko et al., 1998; U.S. Army SBCCOM, 1999).

TABLE 4-4 Evolution of Performance Requirements for Protective Textiles

Date	Garment	Requirements
1960s	XXCC3 underwear	7 days wear 6 hours protection
1970s	CPOG	14 days wear 6 hours protection
1980s	OG84/BDO	22 days wear 24 hours protection
1990s	JSLIST	45 days wear 24 hours protection
2000s	JSLIST P31	60 days wear 24 hours protection
Army After Next	ICS	indefinite wear self-decontamination

Source: Brandler, 1998.

The combination of nanofiber and microfiber or regular multifilament fibers is a new program being initiated in the Drexel-Akron project of the Army Multidisciplinary University Research Initiative (MURI). Although a wide range of properties can be engineered into a fiber, the technology for processing nanofibers in traditional textile machines is not well established. In theory, the nanofibers would provide less resistance to air movement and greater surface area for absorption of gaseous contaminant per unit weight of nanofiber material compared to absorbers based on conventional carbon-fiber technology (Gibson and Schreuder-Gibson, 1999). Neither the dynamic interaction between nanofibers and machine surfaces nor the problems that will be encountered in chemical and mechanical finishing of fabrics containing nanofibers (e.g., snagging, adhesion, melting, agglomeration) have been investigated (ARO, 1997; Gibson and Reneker, 1998).

The durability of the garment can be improved with stronger and tougher fibers and proper design of fabric construction (such as optimization of interlacing density). To improve fabric comfort or reduce heat stress, the permeability and thermal conductivity of the fiber and structure can be increased. Experiments on skin-fabric interactions, results of which could lead to improved performance, can be readily performed. Table 4-5 is a summary of the general improvements in the material properties of fibers that can be made to achieve the design goals for CB protective textiles.

Using clothing to protect an individual from chemical agents can be approached two different ways: (1) by providing an impermeable barrier; or (2) by providing a selectively (semi-)permeable barrier. Materials that create physically impermeable barriers to chemical agents sacrifice the moisture-vapor permeability of the clothing. Although impermeable barrier materials, such as rubber and coated fabrics, allow some degree of moisture-vapor permeability, it is too low to avoid heat stress and thus decreases the wearer's ability to accomplish a mission. Therefore,

TABLE 4-5 Summary of Required Improvements in Fibrous Material Properties

Needs	Properties
Lighter weight	Lower fiber specific gravity
	Lower packing density
Less bulk	Smaller fiber diameter
	Higher packing density
Higher durability	Higher strength, toughness
More comfort	More permeability
Less heat stress	Better thermal conductivity

Source: Ko, 1999.

impermeable materials can only be used effectively for a short time. The impermeable barrier approach was used for protective clothing until the mid-1970s.

Currently, the impermeable barrier approach is used only for gloves, boots, and other special equipment intended for short-term use (such as the suit, contamination avoidance, liquid protection [SCALP] outfit, the toxicological agent protective [TAP] outfit, and the self-contained toxic environment protective outfit [STEPO]).

The newer approach is to use a semipermeable fabric and a sorptive layer that can filter out/decompose chemical agents or to use selectively permeable membrane materials. Sorption can be achieved by using carbon powder or carbon fibers. Carbon powder can be disseminated as foam, as coating on fibers, as filling in hollow fibers, or as part of meltblown fibers. Activated carbon fibers can be used as nonwoven, flocked fabrics or laminated structures. Protection by chemical decomposition of the agents can be achieved by the use of reactive resins or reactive enzymes. The selectively permeable membrane concept is currently under development at the SBCCOM Soldier Systems Center at Natick, Massachusetts (see Figure 4-1).

The BDO consists of a coat and trousers, usually worn over the duty uniform. The BDO has an outer layer of 7-oz/yd^2 of a nylon/cotton blended twill (woodland camouflage) or 6-oz/yd^2 of nylon/cotton/Kevlar twill (desert camouflage) in a twist weave construction. The inner layer consists of activated charcoal impregnated into approximately 90-mil polyurethane foam laminated to a 2-oz/yd^2 nylon tricot liner (Figure 4-2). The inner layer components are laminated together; the top layer essentially floats and is put on as the garment is manufactured. Because of the heavy impregnation of charcoal, some charcoal may be deposited on the skin and clothing under the BDO. The BDO is water resistant, but not waterproof. It provides 24 hours of protection against chemical agents

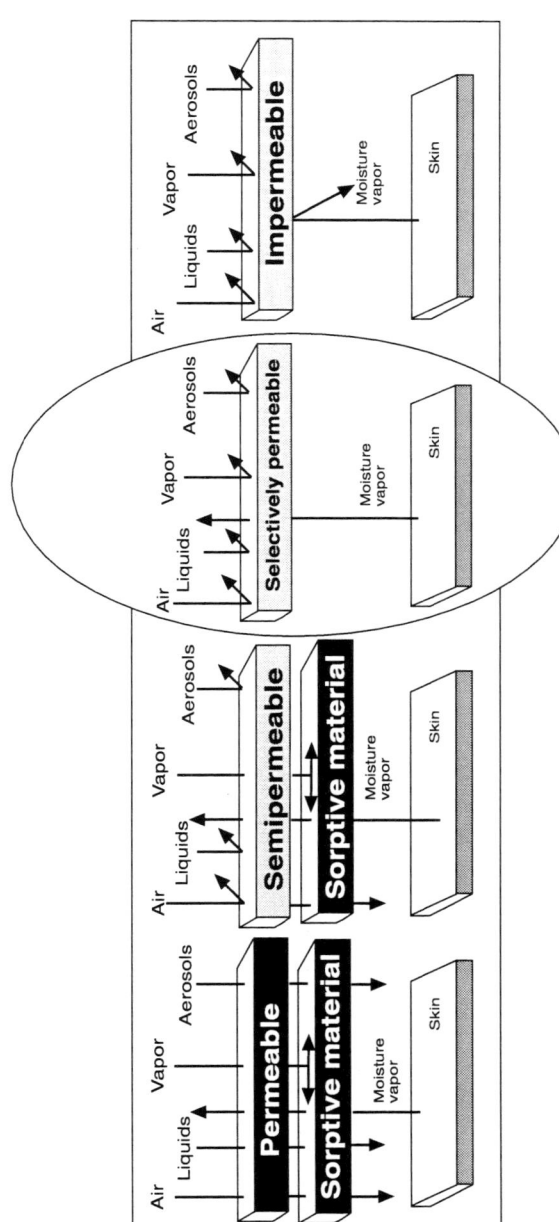

FIGURE 4-1 Construction of a selectively permeable barrier.

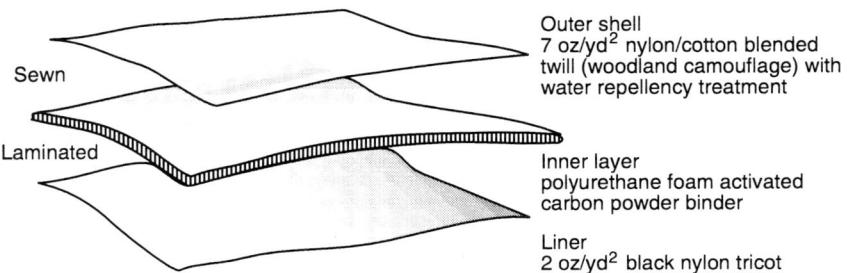

FIGURE 4-2 Components of a typical current barrier system.

once contaminated and has a field durability of 22 days (U.S. Army Office of the Surgeon General, 1997). The BDO's shelf life is 14 years if the packaging is intact.

The Saratoga overgarment (OG84/BDO) was developed for the Marines, who were dissatisfied with the BDO (Mellian, 1999). The Saratoga overgarment is designed for 30 days of continuous wear and provides 24 hours of protection against chemical agent vapors, aerosols, droplets, and all known biological agents. The overgarment consists of an outer layer of cotton ripstop material treated for durability and liquid resistance and an inner filter layer of spherical carbon absorbers laminated between two lightweight polyester materials. The coat features a full-length zippered opening covered by a single protective flap, an integrated hood, hook and pile sleeve closures, and trousers with adjustable waist tabs, suspenders, and closures on the lower outside section of each leg. The Saratoga overgarment can be worn over the duty uniform or directly over undergarments. Advantages of the Saratoga overgarment over the BDO include launderability, lower thermal burden, an extended wearlife, a 15 to 20 year shelf life, and a higher degree of comfort and durability.

JSLIST, the first of a three-phase program, was created to consolidate the programs of individual services to obtain a family of garments and ensembles to meet joint service needs[2] at the lowest practical cost. The

---

[2]The requirements generation system produces information for decision makers on the projected mission needs of the warfighter. The generation of requirements consists of four phases: definition, documentation, validation, and approval. The process evolves from a mission needs statement (MNS) to a capstone requirements document (if applicable) through operational requirements documents. The MNS is a continuing process that normally begins with a review of the latest national security policy, national military strategy, defense planning guidance, joint intelligence guidance, and projected threats and is generated in coordination with the applicable services and agencies, CINCs, and higher headquarters (Chairman of the Joint Chiefs of Staff, 1997).

JSLIST ensemble affords CB protection with reduced physiological heat burden and better integration with weapons systems than previous technologies. The ensemble consists of five clothing items: (1) overgarment, (2) undergarment, (3) duty uniform, (4) boots, and (5) gloves. To date, only two of the five components (the chemical protective overgarment and the multipurpose overboot [MULO]) have been type classified. The remaining items, as well as minor design modifications to the JSLIST overgarment, are being addressed in the JSLIST Pre-Planned Product Improvement (P3I) program.

Procurement for the JSLIST overgarment began in FY 1997. The JSLIST overgarment, which has a shelf life of 15 years, is designed to provide 24-hour chemical protection for 45 days of wear and six launderings. It can be worn over the battledress uniform (BDU) or as a primary garment over underwear, depending on the environment and mission. The overgarment is a two-piece, front-opening garment that has an integral hood, bellow-type pockets, high-waist trousers, adjustable suspenders, and an adjustable waistband. The material is a combination of a nylon/cotton outershell over the Saratoga filter cloth.

The JSLIST has many advantages over the BDO. It can be laundered more often (i.e., less time between washings) and more times; the outer shell materials are stronger and more durable; the sorptive liner materials are cleaner and more breathable; the integrated hood increases the protection capabilities of the suit; the raglan sleeve allows more freedom of movement; the integrated suspenders allow for optimal individual fitting; and lighter weight reduces heat stress.

In addition to improving the ratio of work to rest time, JSLIST garments are designed to be more accurately sized, fitted, and worn by both male and female service personnel. The garments have a seven-size system, in which the coat and trousers are packaged separately. (For logistical reasons, the Navy will only be using a five-size system.) An evaluation of the design, size, and fit of these components revealed that the coat retention cord kept the coat from separating from the trousers at the waistline, but 68 percent of the test participants complained that the cord was uncomfortable (Mellian, 1997). To alleviate the discomfort, the cord was lengthened and modified to be convertible so that it could be unhooked at MOPP 1, MOPP 2, and MOPP 3 levels. Complaints were also registered regarding irritation from the hook-and-pile fasteners at the hood/neck area. Modifications were made to the fasteners, but complaints were still common. It was suggested that research be conducted during the next phase of the JSLIST program to find a softer hook fastener tape (Mellian, 1997).

The JSLIST P3I overgarment program is a follow-on to the JSLIST program. The goal of the JSLIST P3I program is to incorporate mature fabric technologies that have been developed for civilian use into the existing JSLIST design. The program's goals include the development of a 60-day flame-resistant (FR) overgarment, a 30-day FR overgarment, a 30-day FR duty uniform, a 7-day FR overgarment, a 7-day FR undergarment, and a multipurpose protective sock (MPS). Operational and technical tests are being conducted on materials identified through a screening process, and a technology insertion decision is scheduled for the first quarter of FY 2000.

After extended wear, the MPS will provide 12 hours of protection against 10 g/m^2 liquid agent and 5,000 $mg\text{-}min/m^3$ vapor/aerosols if worn under a boot made of permeable material. It also must be comfortable, fit well, be compatible with all Special Operations Forces footwear, and retain its chemical protection after four launderings.

According to requirements, the lightweight chemical/biological protective garment (LCBPG) of the JSLIST P3I program will be designed to provide 6 hours of protection against 10 g/m^2 liquid agent and 5,000 $mg\text{-}min/m^3$ vapor/aerosols for 7 days of field wear in all geographical areas (U.S. Marine Corps, 1999a). The garment will not have to be launderable, but it must weigh no more than four pounds and have a maximum package size of 500 in^3. It is hoped that the LCBPG, which may be worn as an overgarment or as a primary garment over underwear depending on the environment or mission, will reduce the physiological heat burden of the BDO by at least 20 percent.

The JSLIST P3I 60-day overgarment is a joint requirement and will be worn as an overgarment for the BDU or as a primary garment over personal underwear depending on the environment and mission. According to requirements, it will provide 24 hours of protection for 60 days of field wear in all geographical environments. It must retain its chemical protection after eight launderings, weigh less than four pounds, and, like the LCBPG, reduce the physiological heat burden of the BDO.

The JSLIST P3I 30-day overgarment, an Air Force requirement, is similar to the JSLIST P3I 60-day overgarment, but it only has to provide protection for 30 days of field wear and must retain its chemical protection for only four launderings. It will be worn as an overgarment for the duty uniform or as a primary garment over underwear.

The vapor protective undergarment (VPU) is a Special Operations Forces requirement of interest to the Army, Air Force, and Marine Corps, which would provide 12 hours of protection against 10 g/m^2 liquid agent and 10,000 $mg\text{-}min/m^3$ vapor/aerosols for 30 days of field wear. It must retain its chemical protection after four launderings, weigh less than three pounds, and reduce the heat stress burden imposed by the current chemical protective undergarment (CPU).

The Marine Corps has a requirement (also of interest to the Army, Air

Force and Special Operations Forces) for a duty uniform that would enhance existing capability with a lighter, less thermally burdening ensemble. It would be worn by all Marines, except aircrews with special environmental or equipment interface requirements and personnel who deal with large volumes of liquid contaminants.

The joint service protective aircrew ensemble (JPACE) will provide below-the-neck protection against chemical and biological agents for rotary and fixed-wing aircrews. It will be used by all of the services and will replace the Navy/Marine Corps MK-1 undergarment, the Army ABDU-BDO system, and the Air Force CWU-66/P overgarment. Requirements for the ensemble include a 30-day wear time, launderability, compatibility with aircrew-mounted aviation life-support systems, ejection safety, and water survivability. The JPACE will be jointly tested and fielded with the joint service aviation mask and will use JSLIST and JSLIST P3I materials, designs, and documentation to the maximum extent possible. Separate garments may be considered for fixed-wing and rotary-wing aircrews.

Masks

The respiratory system is the most vulnerable human system to airborne contaminants. Some estimates for organic vapors are that 10 to 1,000 times more vapor is absorbed through the lungs than through the skin (e.g., Leung and Paustenbach, 1994). The gas exchange region of an adult's respiratory system has a surface area of 75 m^2 to 100 m^2, 40 times that of the skin, and is in direct contact with the external environment. This surface is also the thinnest membrane in the body so gases can readily diffuse through it. Thus, for many chemical contaminants, including nonvesicant chemical warfare agents, other routes of absorption are only important when the respiratory system is well protected.

Because of the importance and extreme vulnerability of the respiratory system, humans have evolved extensive natural defense mechanisms for protecting it from environmental insults. These include mechanisms in the nose, throat, and conductive airways and a system of branching tubes that conduct air to the gas exchange region to protect the more sensitive gas exchange, or alveolar, region from chemicals at low concentrations and from chemicals with low acute toxicity. These defenses cannot, however, protect against the highly toxic and rapidly acting chemical warfare agents to which deployed forces may be exposed. For these reasons, respiratory protection is a major component in the contamination avoidance doctrine, and respirators of various types have been developed and fielded.

A respirator can be defined as a covering over the mouth and nose that protects the respiratory system by reducing the amount of airborne contaminant inhaled. The two basic classes of respirators are "air-purifying" respirators and "atmosphere-supplying" respirators. The former uses lung power to draw air through a filter and into the respirator. Because the mask is under negative pressure with respect to the external environment during inhalation, facial seals must be tight to ensure protection. Atmosphere-supplying respirators rely on the delivery of clean air from another environment via an air line or compressed air tank. These respirators keep the mask under positive pressure at all times and thus prevent inward leakage of contaminated air.

Respirators differ in the types and levels of protection they provide and the degree of encumbrance they impose. Other factors that affect the level of protection include the growth of facial hair, the shape of the wearer's face, the fit, material inconsistencies, adverse reactions to adhesives or sealants, and potential incompatibility with night vision goggles.

Half-face respirators are the simplest and least encumbering. They cover the nose and mouth and seal across the bridge of the nose and under the chin. They are characterized by light weight, comfort, moderate to good filter efficiency, and the ability to speak and be understood. However, these disposable respirators provide no eye protection, which can be critical for some agents, and seal poorly against the face. Half-face respirators are similar to the masks physicians wear in an operating room. A variation of these simple respirators is the cartridge, elastomeric, half-mask respirator that covers the nose and mouth, fits and seals better, has inhalation and exhalation valves, and can accommodate different types of cartridges for different contaminants. They do not protect the eyes, however, and, therefore, do not meet the protection factor (PF) required for typical biological threats.

The full face-piece respirator protects the eyes, provides a better seal against the face than the half-mask, may include a speaking diaphragm, and may have an inner mask to control the flow of inhaled air to reduce lens fogging and dead volume. Some masks are attached by a flexible tube to an oversized cartridge worn on the belt or chest; others have a single filter cartridge located on one side to facilitate aiming a weapon. Most military masks are full face-piece respirators with an inner mask and a speaking diaphragm. Current U.S. masks (e.g., M40) are designed to use NATO standard filter canisters. In addition, masks must be capable of being combined with other protective clothing as part of a fully integrated protective suit, and they must provide laser and ballistic fragmentation eye protection.

Forced air-purifying respirators supply clean air through a hose. They may be used with half-mask or full face-piece masks or with a hood or helmet. They maintain a positive pressure in the mask at all times and eliminate the effort required to draw air through a filter. They provide a higher level of protection than cartridge respirators, but current versions are heavier and more cumbersome than cartridge units and require either portable air compressors and larger filter units or must be coupled to compressed air tanks. The tank-equipped self-contained breathing apparatus does not restrict mobility and can be used in low-oxygen situations. A two-stage regulator maintains positive pressure in the mask at all times.

Oxygen "rebreather" systems are sealed systems that recycle expired air. They use carbon dioxide scrubbers and add small amounts of pure oxygen to replace the oxygen removed during breathing. They have longer service life than tanked compressed air, but the mask may be under negative pressure creating a risk of fire or explosion from the use of oxygen and possible leaks of the strongly caustic materials used for carbon dioxide scrubbing if water gets into the system (e.g., during decontamination operations).

An intermediate category of respirators is the powered air-purifying respirator, which uses battery-powered pumps to draw air through a filter and delivers it under positive pressure to the mask (either half-mask or full face-piece). The pump can be carried on the belt or mounted on the apparatus in a fixed location. These devices can provide a high level of protection because the mask is under positive pressure, and they reduce the effort required for breathing. However, they are heavy, have battery life limitations, and cannot be used in an oxygen deficient atmosphere.

Level of Protection. The level of protection provided by a respirator is characterized by a protection factor, *PF*, which is the ratio of the external concentration of contaminant to the contamination level inside the mask.

$$PF = \frac{concentration\ outside\ mask}{concentration\ inside\ mask}$$

Thus a *PF* of 1 represents no protection, and a *PF* of 100 means the wearer's exposure is reduced by a factor of 100. Ideally, the PF will be greater than 10,000. The technical requirements for military protective masks require that they provide a PF 1,667 for 88 percent of the population, a PF 6,667 for 75 percent of the population, and a PF 10,000 for 68 percent of the population (Kirkwood, 1998). Nevertheless, even if properly functioning, contamination can enter by three possible routes: through the filter, through leaks in the facial seal, or through the exhalation valve. Leakage in the facial seal is the most common source of exposure in current masks (Hinds, 1999).

The weakest link in respirator performance is the quality of the facial seal, or fit of the respirator on the face. Because everyone's face is shaped differently, the fit of masks is often less than ideal; fit can also be adversely affected by the growth of facial hair. Full face-piece masks provide a better fit for a wider range of faces than half-face masks.

Three levels of tests can be used to evaluate fit. The simplest and least precise is subjective "fit checks," such as negative pressure tests and positive pressure tests. These tests are used every time the mask is donned to verify that it is properly seated on the face and is operating properly. In the negative pressure test, the wearer blocks the filter inlets with the palms of the hands and tries to suck the mask down against the face. If it can be held against the face, it passes the test; if not, it fails. In the positive pressure test, the wearer blocks the exhalation valve and tries to exhale to sense any leakage. These tests give only a gross evaluation of fit but do warn the wearer of a malfunction.

The next two levels of tests are used to determine which respirator type or size fits an individual best. Qualitative fit tests are also subjective pass/fail tests but include tests of respirator function, as well as fit. The wearer tests whether a vapor is smelled when the mask is equipped with activated charcoal cartridges and whether an irritant smoke is detectable when the mask is equipped with high-efficiency filters.

The most precise tests are quantitative fit tests, which, as the name suggests, provide a quantitative measure of fit. One test involves wearing a respirator with high-efficiency filters in a test aerosol environment and measuring the aerosol concentrations inside the respirator (by means of a probe through the respirator body) and outside the respirator. A fit factor (FF) is calculated from the ratio of these two quantities.

$$FF = \frac{outside\ concentration}{inside\ concentration\ (filter\ penetration = 0)}$$

Test aerosols include corn oil and sodium chloride and naturally occurring condensation nuclei. Another test measures leakage flow rate for a controlled negative pressure in the mask. Typical equipment can measure fit factors from 1 to 10,000, or even 100,000.

An example of a quantitative fit test is the M41 protection assessment test system, a small portable instrument designed to quantitatively validate the fit of the face piece (U.S. Army SBCCOM, 1999). This test instrument, based on a miniature condensation nucleus counter, continuously samples and counts microscopic particles both inside and outside the mask and calculates a fit factor. The Army, Marine Corps, and Air Force are fielding this test system for use with the M40, M42, and MCU-2/P series masks; the Navy is evaluating it for use with its MCU-2/P series masks (DoD, 1999).

against petroleum, oils, and lubricants, as well as providing flame resistance. The sole is designed to provide traction on various surfaces, including dirt and metal. Key requirements for the MULO are to provide 24 hours of protection against 10 g/m² challenge by all liquid agents; resistance to incidental splashing by petroleum, oils, and lubricants; self-extinguishing flame resistance; 60 days wear in all geographical areas without degradation of protection; and the capability of being decontaminated to an operationally safe level using standard decontaminants. Improvements of this boot over the previous GVO/BVO include more durability, lighter weight, and better CB protection (DoD, 1998b).

Barrier Creams

Barrier creams are designed to prevent or reduce the penetration and absorption of hazardous materials into the skin, thus preventing skin lesions and other toxic effects from dermal exposure. Moisturizers, which are frequently used to treat "dry" skin, as well as to maintain healthy skin, may have common characteristics and ingredients with barrier creams (Zhai and Maibach, 1998). Barrier creams could solve a number of persistent percutaneous problems by: (1) mitigating the consequences of partial closures, (2) providing early protection while protective gear is being donned, and (3) permitting transition from Mask-Only to MOPP 4 status. An ideal barrier cream would be nonirritating, nonallergenic for contact dermatitis, non-photo irritating, non-photoallergenic for contact dermatitis, nonflammable, and not likely to cause contact urticaria syndrome.

The effect of a barrier cream may depend on the dermatopharmacokinetic (DPK) properties of the chemical challenge and other factors (Packham et al., 1994; Wigger-Alberti et al., 1997). A current limitation of barrier creams is that they must be applied in large doses (e.g., 0.15 mm thickness), which could interfere with the physiological mechanisms of the skin (see Chapters 5 and 6 and Appendix C for more details).

Impacts on Effectiveness

Tests and real-world experiences with PPEs have revealed numerous shortcomings. Depending on the outside temperature and the level of work, MOPP postures above MOPP 0 can result in the following performance limitations:

- speech and communications problems
- impaired hearing
- reduced vision (e.g., acuity, field of view, depth perception)

- difficulty recognizing other individuals in MOPP
- heat injuries
- dehydration
- inadequate nutrition
- combat stress
- mood swings and claustrophobia
- impaired thinking and judgment
- reduced manual dexterity

In recent years, the impacts of the effects of wearing MOPP on combat operations have been studied extensively during combined arms exercises, field exercises, and laboratory studies. Dugway Proving Ground, for example, has administered the Chemical Biological (CB) Contact Point and Test Program (Project DO49) to quantify the effects of wearing protective clothing on the performance of military tasks. This program has five operational areas: maintenance operations, night reconnaissance operations, missile operations, armor operations, and signal operations. The following observations are examples of the decrements that have been found:

- In a variety of tasks, degradation was 20 to 50 percent (U.S. Army, 1987).
- Time to complete tasks increased (Chow et al., 1998).
- Oxygen consumption increased about 10 percent in full PPE compared to in light clothes, indicating that personnel in MOPP 4 must use more energy than personnel in MOPP 0 to perform the same tasks (U.S. Army, 1991b).
- Reduced sensory awareness made it harder for personnel to stay awake when tired (Joint Chiefs of Staff, 1995).
- Soldiers required one-and-one-half to three times longer to perform tasks requiring manual dexterity in MOPP 4 than without PPE (U.S. Army, 1991b).
- Performing a task for the first time took longer, as much as 30 percent longer in MOPP 4 (Gawron et al., 1998; U.S. Army, 1987).
- Troops tended to omit or perform certain tasks poorly (e.g., camouflage and support activities) (U.S. Army, 1986).
- The performance levels for cognitive tasks was lower (Kelly et al., 1988; Taylor and Orlansky, 1993; U.S. Army, 1991b; Williams et al., 1995). In one instance, encoding decreased by almost 23 percent (U.S. Army, 1991b).
- Leader performance declined (e.g., they became exhausted, slept less, became disoriented or lost, became irritable, and delegated less authority) (U.S. Army, 1986; 1994).

PHYSICAL PROTECTION

- Leaders were often the first MOPP casualties (U.S. Army, 1986).
- Unit movement formations tended to bunch up (perhaps to help leaders maintain control) (U.S. Army, 1992).
- When platoon leaders became casualties, it took four times as long for a MOPP 4 platoon to realize it was leaderless than an unencumbered platoon. The next senior soldier assumed command 85 percent less often than in non-PPE exercises (U.S. Army, 1986).
- PPE overboots provided poor footing on hilly terrain, loose ground, and wet ground (U.S. Army, 1992).
- PPE garments absorbed rain and became very heavy and cumbersome (U.S. Army, 1992).
- Rifle marksmanship dropped 15 to 19 percent for soldiers in MOPP 4 (U.S. Army, 1991b).
- Individual weapon-firing rates decreased 20 percent in defensive actions and 40 percent in offensive actions. It took twice as long and nearly twice as many soldiers to complete an attack (U.S. Army, 1986).
- The proportion of enemy personnel engaged decreased by one-third (U.S. Army, 1986).
- Weapon crews used terrain much less effectively for cover and concealment, and the number of casualties suffered per enemy defender killed increased by 75 percent (U.S. Army, 1986).
- Units in MOPP 4 tended to take greater risks, especially light and dismounted infantry (e.g., using easier routes and closer formations, not always sterilizing kill zones before crossing) (U.S. Army, 1994).
- Shots fired at friendly instead of enemy soldiers increased from 5 to almost 20 percent (U.S. Army, 1986).
- Indirect fire support was less responsive because artillery and mortar units sacrificed time for accuracy (U.S. Army, 1994). There was also a tendency to use less direct fire and more indirect fire (e.g., platoons called for three times more indirect fire). Indirect fire was more effective than individual weapons in inflicting casualties on the enemy (U.S. Army, 1986).
- Land navigation was seriously degraded (e.g., disorientation and bunching up of armored, mechanized, and dismounted soldiers), particularly at night (U.S. Army, 1994).
- Night vision devices could not be used while personnel were wearing masks (U.S. Army, 1992).
- Radio communication was difficult because of reduced clarity and volume (U.S. Army, 1992). The voicemitter made speakers sound brassy and muffled, and consonants were blurred. The hood and

background noise (e.g., from breathing, garment movement, etc.) degraded hearing (U.S. Army, 1991b).
- Communications were only about half as effective as in a non-PPE environment. Total time spent on radio traffic more than doubled. The number and length of radio transmissions rose by 50 percent (U.S. Army, 1986).
- Time to chart positions in a shipboard combat information center degraded by approximately 24 percent (Garrison et al., 1982).
- Recognition and identification of soldiers and leaders in MOPP 3 and MOPP 4 were difficult because the usual visual cues were hidden (U.S. Army, 1994).
- Logistics operations took longer and became confused (U.S. Army, 1994).
- Maintenance took longer, in one study about 30 percent longer (Shipton et al., 1988).
- Recovering armored vehicles took up to 20 percent longer; repairing weapons took up to 70 percent longer (U.S. Army, 1994).
- Performance of projected sortie generation capability decreased with increasing levels of individual protection (Gawron et al., 1998).
- Target acquisition was more difficult because the field of view was reduced and hearing was restricted (U.S. Army, 1994).
- Movements, maneuvers, and fire support were harder to synchronize, and many tasks took longer to perform (e.g., rates of march decreased significantly and led to increased fuel usage) (U.S. Army, 1994).
- Under some conditions, performance degraded significantly within one hour, although endurance could be extended by adjusting the ambient temperature, amount of drinking water, and/or frequency of rest periods (Taylor and Orlansky, 1993).

Reviews of studies on the effects of PPE on performance in the other services support many of these findings. However, there are problems associated with many of these studies. For example, some of the studies cited above tested out-of-date clothing system components, and these results cannot be directly extended to performance while wearing newer components of the ensemble. Also, there can be different interpretations of the same data, and it is also difficult to conclude that the findings apply to all types of tasks. This suggests that additional research is needed to determine how performance can be improved, with changes in the protective ensemble, to increase the likelihood that U.S. forces can successfully prosecute their missions in a CB environment. (For comprehensive reviews, see, for example, Carr et al., 1980a, 1980b; DoD, 1997b; Draper and Lombardi, 1986; Goldman et al., 1981; Rakaczky, 1981; Taylor and Orlansky, 1987, 1991, 1993.)

Patient Protective Equipment

As of early 1999, only three items of patient protective equipment had been fielded: the patient protective wrap, the decontaminable litter, and the resuscitation device individual chemical (RDIC). R&D on new equipment, especially in the private sector, is continuing as needs continue to be identified.

Patient Protective Wrap

Because the treatment of chemical casualties often requires removal of the PPE and precludes donning of replacement garments, a patient protective wrap has been developed. The wrap, which is designed to be used once and then discarded, is sturdy, lightweight (approximately 2.7 kg), and protects the patient from all known chemical agents for up to six continuous hours. There is a transparent window on the top sheet of the wrap and protective sleeves for passing through intravenous tubing.

The wrap is designed to be used on a litter, but, if necessary, can be used as a field litter. It is recommended, but not required, that the patient wear a mask while in the wrap. However, cardboard inserts must be placed in the wrap before the casualty to hold the window material away from the patient's face. Although the wrap is permeable to oxygen and carbon dioxide, because the rate at which typical patients produce carbon dioxide is slightly faster than the rate at which it passes through the wrap, the carbon dioxide levels slowly build up inside the wrap. Therefore, patients may not remain in the wrap for more than six hours.

Decontaminable Litter

Canvas litters, traditionally used to transport casualties after exposure to liquid blister agents, have been found to continue to desorb vapors for 72 hours after all surface contaminants were removed. This problem led to the development of a litter made of monofilament polypropylene, which has high tensile strength and low elasticity. The fabric, a honeycomb weave through which liquid passes easily, does not absorb liquid chemical agents, is not degraded by current decontaminating solutions, is flame retardant, is rip resistant, and is treated to withstand exposure to weather and sunlight. The litter has retractable handles and a metal pole frame. The metal parts have been painted with chemical agent resistant coating paint.

Resuscitation Device, Individual Chemical

The RDIC is a ventilation system consisting of a compressible butyl rubber bag, a NATO standard C_2 canister filter, a nonrebreathing valve, a cricothyroid cannula adapter, and a flexible hose connected to an oropharyngeal mask. The butyl rubber bag resists penetration of liquid chemical agent and can be decontaminated easily. There will be one RDIC for each air ambulance, one for each ground ambulance, and one at each chemical agent medical treatment facility.

Summary

Current R&D on PPE is addressing the continuing problems with JSLIST, including leaks around joints and seals; reduced, but still significant, heat loading problems; weight and bulk problems; and difficulty with decontamination and reuse. Future enhancements in textiles and fabrics could include (1) integrated detection capability to alert the wearer to the presence of contamination and to indicate the time remaining at the highest protection level, and (2) the use of advanced solid sorbents with improved properties over charcoal materials.

With the current design of the mask and the JSLIST overgarment, during the transition from Mask-Only to MOPP 4 status, the mask seal may be momentarily broken. If troops are in an area of high agent concentration, this momentary breach could result in incapacitation or death. All masks have potential problems with leakage around seals due to improper fit, the growth of facial hair, and material inconsistencies. Available technology for regenerating filters and adsorbents has not advanced greatly in the past few years, and adsorbent saturation limit the mask's effective use time. Gloves are cumbersome, reduce tactile efficiency, and don't integrate well with weapons (i.e., trigger guards on rifles, etc.). Boots are heavy and uncomfortable, and extended wear can cause dermatological problems. Barrier creams are being investigated and evaluated for use in combat.

COLLECTIVE PROTECTION

Risks, Challenges, and Requirements

CPE provides a relatively unencumbered safe environment in which eating, surgery, and other activities can be performed. Collective protective systems have been developed as stand-alone structures or overpressurized (i.e., positive pressure) vehicles and vans. Ideally, this equipment could protect against physical as well as CB threats. However, current collective protection equipment is vulnerable to physical threats, such as shrapnel and projectiles, cannot be erected easily, and is rarely available (DoD, 1999; Institute for Defense Analyses, 1999). Protection against physical threats has been sacrificed for portability.

The major challenges for stand-alone collective protective systems are availability, portability, functionality, and integrity of the barrier. Functionality includes ingress and egress that minimize or eliminate the possibility of internal contamination. Challenges for protecting crews in vehicles include integrating collective protection measures into vehicle designs. Improved protection in any environment depends on filtration and adsorbent technologies, as well as the availability of protective equipment. The number of collective protective units available for deployment is much lower than the number required for most activities in a large-scale CB environment.

Filters

The M48/M48A1 is a 100 ft^3/min filter currently used in the M1A1/A2 Abrams tank, M93 modular collective protection equipment (MCPE), CB protected shelter, and the paladin self-propelled howitzer. The M56 is a 200-ft^3/min filter currently used as the basic filter set in the MCPE and in naval applications. M56 filters can be stacked for higher airflow rates. 600 ft^3/min and 1,200 ft^3/min stainless steel fixed installation gas filters are currently used for fixed-sites where high volumes of airflow are required. They can be stacked to provide higher airflow rates.

Filter Systems

M8A3 Gas Particulate Filter Unit (GPFU)

The M8A3 GPFU is a 12-ft^3/min system that provides air to the M42A1/A2 armored vehicle crewman ventilated face mask. It is also used in the Army's M113 armored personnel carrier variants and the Marine Corps' AAVP7A1 amphibious vehicle.

M13A1 GPFU

The M13A1 GPFU is a 20-ft^3/min system that provides air to the M42A1/A2 armored vehicle crewmen ventilated face masks. It is also used on the M1A1/A2 Abrams tanks, Bradley fighting vehicles, MLRS, tank transporter, and other vehicles.

Recirculation Filter Blowers

Recirculation filter blowers are used to eliminate the risks of residual contamination through a 600 ft^3/min continuous air-filtration cycle. These blowers are portable, self-contained, and equipped with replaceable filters. They are used with the M28 and M20A1 shelter systems. The filter life can be as long as 2,000 hours depending on the contamination level (Gander, 1997).

Intellitec Biochemical Filter Blower Unit (BFBU)

The BFBU is designed to provide filtered air and overpressure to the ground-based common sensor-heavy, the XM4 command and control vehicle, and the armored treatment and transport vehicle. The BFBU can be operated in the bypass mode, the low-flow NBC mode, and the high-flow NBC mode. In nonthreat conditions, the bypass mode delivers 100 to 140 ft^3/min of make-up air and filters dust through a two-stage filtration system. The NBC modes use two standard M48 or M48A1 gas/particulate filters with precleaners and can be set at up to 140 ft^3/min in the low-flow mode and 210 ft^3/min in the high-flow mode. The unit can monitor the overpressure and can be switched between the high-flow and low-flow modes either manually or automatically on receipt of an alarm signal to maintain required overpressure at the minimum current draw. The control electronics monitor the pressure drop across the filter by delivering an analogue signal that drives an external display, allowing the occupants to monitor filter status (Gander, 1997).

Filter Residual Life Indicator

The filter residual life indicator detects an adsorption wave within the carbon bed of the filter to monitor the residual absorption capacity of in-service activated carbon air purification devices. The detector technology consists of a chemoselective polymer-coated surface acoustic wave (SAW) device. The polymer coating sorbs agent and causes a shift in signal frequency. The specificity of the coating allows for selectivity towards CB agents. This device is small (approximately 1 cm^2), has a high sensitivity, gives a rapid response, and only costs $3.00 (Katz, 1990; Morrison, 1998) but has not yet been fielded.

Protective Structures and Systems

Currently Fielded Structures and Systems

M51 Protective Shelter. The M51 protective shelter is a trailer-mounted system that is used primarily by battalion aid stations and other medical units but can also be used as a temporary rest and relief shelter. It consists of a 10-man shelter, a protective entrance, and a support system. The shelter and protective entrance support themselves through air-filled ribs. The protective entrance minimizes carryover of vapor contamination from outside the shelter and paces entries to the shelter to prevent loss of shelter overpressure. The air-handling system, which is permanently mounted in the trailer, provides filtered, environmentally conditioned air. This system can be erected by four to six people in approximately one hour. The M51 was found to be unsuitable by users because of excessive weight, excessive set-up time, insufficient usable floor space, insufficient throughput of medical patients, lack of natural ventilation and lighting, and lack of space on transport vehicles (DoD, 1999; Siegel, 1998; U.S. Army and U.S. Marine Corps, 1992).

M20A1/M28 Simplified Collective Protective Equipment. The simplified collective protective equipment is used to convert an interior room of an existing structure into a positive overpressure, NBC collective protection shelter for command, control, and communications, medical treatment, and soldier relief. The M20A1 is a room liner for existing shelters, and the M28 is a liner for the tent expandable modular personnel (TEMPER). The simplified collective protective equipment consists of a CB vapor-resistant polyethylene liner; a collapsible protective entrance that allows entry to and exit from the protected area; a hermetically sealed filter canister that provides filtered air to both the liner and the protective entrance; and a support kit. The support kit contains ducting, lighting, sealing and repair material, and an electronically-powered blower. A P3I is under way to allow more people to enter at one time and protect hospitals under tents. It will also provide liquid agent resistant liners, protective liners for tents, interconnectors, and an interface with environmental control units (DoD, 1999; U.S. Army and U.S. Marine Corps, 1992).

Chemically Protected Deployable Medical System (CP DEPMEDS). The chemically protected deployable medical system will provide environmentally controlled collective protection for field hospitals. Users will be able to perform medical treatment in a CB environment to sustain a 72-hour mission. The protection is provided through the integration of M28 simplified collective protective equipment; chemically protected air conditioners, heaters, water distribution, and latrines; and alarm systems. CB resistant gaskets replace the existing shelter seals in the DEPMEDS ISO shelter. The field deployable environmental control unit provides air conditioning, and the Army space heater provides heating. Both are protected through the addition of a CB kit. Initial operational capability is projected for the second quarter of fiscal year 2001 (DoD, 1999; Siegel, 1998).

Portable Collective Protection System. The portable collective protection system was developed by the Marines to provide an uncontaminated, positive-pressure shelter for use as a command and control facility or a rest and relief facility. The shelter holds 12 to 14 people at a time and can be erected within 30 minutes by four people wearing MOPP 4 gear. The system includes a protective shelter, a support kit, and a hermetically sealed filter canister. The shelter consists of a tent and fly, and is divided into a main area and two smaller compartments, an entry area, and a storage area. The tent floor and fly are made of a saranaex composite material. An airlock allows for decontamination of entering personnel and for purging of chemical agent vapors. The support kit contains a motor/blower assembly that supplies air to the system and flexible ducts that guide the air to the hermetically sealed filter canister and then to the shelter. The hermetically sealed aluminum canister contains a gas filter and a particulate filter (DoD, 1999; U.S. Marine Corps, 1999b).

RDT&E Programs for Collective Protective Systems and Structures

Chemically and Biologically Protected Shelter. The chemically and biologically protected shelter is designed to provide a contamination-free, environmentally controlled work area for a battalion aid station moving up to three times a day or a division clearing station moving once every three days. This system will be a direct replacement for the M51 chemically protected shelter. It consists of a dedicated heavy high mobility multipurpose wheeled vehicle, a lightweight multipurpose shelter mounted on the back of the vehicle, a 300 ft^2 airbeam-supported shelter, and a hydraulically powered environmental support system. A high-mobility trailer is towed by the vehicle to transport the medical equipment and a 10kW tactical quiet generator set for auxiliary power. The chemically and biologically protected shelter can transport a crew of four and can be set up or taken down in 20 minutes in a conventional environment and 40 minutes in a CB contaminated environment. The airbeam-supported soft shelter is fabricated of a fluoropolymer/Kevlar laminate that is CB resistant, capable of being decontaminated, environmentally durable, and flame resistant. The chemically and biologically protected shelter can process 10 litter/ambulatory patients per hour in a CB environment. This system is presently in limited production; fielding is scheduled to begin in the fourth quarter of fiscal year 1999 (DoD, 1999; Siegel, 1998; U.S. Army Soldier Systems Center, 1997).

Joint Transportable Collective Protection System. The joint transportable collective protection system will be a modular shelter system that can process contaminated personnel through a contamination control area into a toxic-free area. The system, which will be expandable to meet changing mission needs, will consist of an environmental control unit, a filter/blower, and a power unit and can be used as a stand-alone structure or within existing structures. The system will protect against all CB threat agents, toxic industrial materials, and nuclear/radiological particulate matter for 30 days after initial agent exposure without a filter change. The development program for this system is scheduled to begin in FY 2000 (U.S. Army Soldier Systems Center, 1999).

Advanced Integrated Collective Protection System. The advanced integrated collective protection system is a fully integrated collective protection system designed for installation on tactical vans and shelters. Major system elements include an NBC survivable enclosure, a turbo-diesel engine/alternator, an advanced air filtration system, an environmental control unit, and a system control unit. It uses a deep-bed carbon vapor filter system for extended gas filter life. The filtration system has a mission life more than twice that of any filtration system currently in use. The combined components provide reductions in overall size, weight, and energy and eliminate the need for additional electrical power from the host system (DoD, 1999; Negron, 1998).

Modular Collective Protection Equipment (100-, 200-, 400-, 600-ft^3/min Systems). The modular collective protection equipment system is a family of equipment designed to provide positive-pressure NBC protection for a variety of vans, vehicles, and shelters. It consists of four different sized filter units, three different free-standing protective entrances, three integral protective entrances, a motor controller, and a static frequency converter. The equipment has common parts and mountings and interchangeable connections and accessories (DoD, 1998b, 1999).

ADVANCED FILTERS AND ADSORBENTS

The key to protection against chemical agents is to remove them from the individual's personal environment. Of the several methods that can be used for removal, trapping, and sometimes deactivating, agent(s) on filters and adsorbing materials is the most practical. Filters and adsorbents are used in filter cartridges for masks and in air purifiers for collective protection systems; adsorbents are also used to impregnate liners for the fabric of the JSLIST chemical protective ensemble. Filters can be improved by modifying fiber structures and by improving the integration of filters into protective systems. Improving the adsorbers in current use will be critical for protecting deployed forces in the future. Therefore, substantial R&D is being done to develop advanced adsorbers that will improve the chemical agent filtration capabilities of current single-pass filter systems as well as regenerative filtration systems (that are under development). Future filter systems with advanced adsorbents will be smaller, lighter weight, and less combustible. So far, some candidate materials have been identified, but complete investigations have not been done on the relationships between adsorption performance and adsorbent properties (e.g., pore structure, surface characteristics, and impregnant reactivity).

Filters

Current air-purification devices have two parts: (1) an aerosol/particulate-matter filter, and (2) a gas absorber. Typical specifications for a military air-purification device for individual protection are listed in Table 4-6 (Kuhlmann, 1998).

The aerosol/particulate-matter filter is built up of layers of glass fibers, and the space between the fibers is large in relation to the size of the aerosol/particulate matter in contaminated air streams. Consequently, a filter of this kind functions by attracting and retaining particles rather than by entrapping them. Attraction/retention is an important factor in protecting against some bioaerosols (e.g., the diameter of the bacteriophage 0-X 174 surrogate for the hepatitis C virus has a diameter of only 27 nm) (ASTM, 1993).

Early laboratory studies showed that porous fiber-type filters could remove 99.998 percent of a bacterial aerosol (Zuykova, 1959); tests of a medical field hospital showed that an ambient challenge as high as 100,000 organisms/ft^3 could be reduced to 0.015 organisms/ft^3 (Landsberg, 1964).

TABLE 4-6 Requirements for the C2 Air-Purification Device

Requirement	Specification
Aerosol efficiency	99.99 @ 32 lpm
Cyanogen chloride gas life	30 min @ 4,000 mg/m^3
Dimethyl methylphosphonate gas life	59 min @ 3,000 mg/m^3

Source: Katz, 1999.

Recent tests on a multistage bioaerosol filtration system at a large metropolitan medical facility showed that the filtration media remained effective after a year of continual operation (Fadem and Tsai, 1998). This system incorporated various aspects of Brownian motion, gravitational field, electrical forces, thermal gradients, turbulent diffusion, and inertial impaction. The microorganism genera found in the internal atmosphere of the facility at levels ranging from 100 to 200 colony-forming units/m^3 included acremonium, actionmycetes, aspergillus, bacillus, chysosporium, clasdosporium, micrococcus, mucor, penicillium, phoma, rhieopus, rhodotorula, staphylococcus, streptococcus, and gram-positive and gram-negative bacteria. Initial airborne fungal and bacterial levels of 187 and 40 colony forming unit per cubic meter were reduced to non-detectable levels after 24 hours of filter operation corresponding to 264 air changes in an 819 ft^3-room. Corona-charged, melt-blown polypropylene media (Electret AEM-1, AEM-2 and AFF-200) exceeded the threshold criteria for emery-oil penetration and pressure drop (Kuhlmann, 1998).

Absorbers

A gas absorber follows the particle filter to remove any gaseous toxic materials in the air stream and/or gases volatilized from particulate material retained by the filter. The gas-absorbing component of the air-purification device consists of activated carbon. Other absorbents have been evaluated, but none was found to be superior to activated carbon in removing chemical agents from contaminated air streams.

Activated carbon is produced by heating charcoal with carbon dioxide or steam at 800° to 1,000°C. The activated product contains numerous pores and cavities for trapping toxic gases in the contaminated air stream. The activated carbon used in most air-purification devices has a surface area of several hundred to more than a thousand m^2/g.

Some low molecular mass chemical agents, such as arsine (agent SA), hydrogen cyanide (agent AC), and cyanogen chloride (agent CK), are not strongly absorbed or retained by activated charcoal. Until recently, an activated carbon formulation containing compounds of copper, silver, and chromium (ASC carbon or Whetlerite) was used to physically absorb and chemically decompose these highly volatile chemical agents. Concerns about the potential inhalation of carbon dust containing carcinogenic hexavalent chromium and failure of the canisters to pass an Environmental Protection Agency submersion test, however, prompted a reformulation of the absorbent (Katz, 1990). The current gas absorber used in military air-purification devices is activated carbon treated with copper, silver, zinc, molybdenum, and triethylenediamine.

This type of bonded activated carbon was found to surpass the minimum CK and dimethyl methylphosphate (DMMP) gas life requirements for the C2 air-purification device (Kuhlmann, 1998). A 100-cm^3, 24-mm deep bonded carbon disc showed a 50 percent-longer-than-threshold-criterion CK gas life and nearly a 2.5-times-longer-than-threshold-criterion DMMP gas life. In addition, the pressure drop for the bonded carbon disc was 9.5 mm of water below the threshold criterion of 22.5 mm of water.

Carbon absorbents prepared from fullerene soot have been reported to be superior to charcoal-based absorbents for adsorbing halocarbons from humid gas streams (Bell et al., 1998). The soot, obtained from pyrolyzing a mixture of Carbon-60–Carbon-70 and higher fullerenes, was blended with a polymeric binder and pressed into discs prior to carbonization in an inert atmosphere. Compared to sorbents prepared from commercial carbon black, pellets from fullerenes had larger surface areas, longer breakthrough times, better dynamic capacities, higher adsorption rate coefficients, and greater transverse crush strength.

The absorption capacities of carbon fiber-based absorbents have been found to be greater than those of granulated activated carbons. The advantages of using fiber-based adsorbents in individual protection air-purification devices would be lower pressure drop, smaller volume, and lower mass. Carbon-loaded nanofibers prepared by electrospinlacing have been proposed for filter use but will have to be tested to demonstrate their applicability to the absorption of toxic gas in individual protection air-purification devices (Schreuder-Gibson, 1998).

Service-Life Indicators

Air-purification devices have finite capacities that limit their service life. A means for determining residual filter life after initial use or after prolonged storage has been and continues to be a subject of active research. Color-change indicators (Lielke et al., 1986) and liquid-crystal sensors (Henderson and Novak, 1992) were among the first approaches taken to monitor residual life. More recently, a SAW chemical sensor has been used to monitor the residual absorption capacity of in-service activated carbon air-purification devices (Dominguez et al., 1998). This small, rugged, sensitive sensor had a large, nonspecific dynamic range. Its surface was prepared with a 50-nm film of fluoropolyol prior to evaluating its ability to sense DMMP and thereby indicate exhaustion of its absorption capacity. The sensor successfully monitored DMMP breakthrough in real time without degrading the performance of the air-purification device.

SAW chemical sensors, as well as semiconductor devices and ion-mobility spectrometry, have been evaluated as filter life-indicator systems for air-purification devices in tanks and other armored vehicles

(Nieuwenhuizen et al., 1998). Ion mobility spectrometry was the most promising.

Regeneration

In the absence of a reliable service life indicator system, schedules for replacement have been developed. Pressure and temperature swing absorption is also being investigated as an alternative. The alternative system would have to be completely regenerable so that the absorbents would not have to be replaced, and the time the air-purification device operates in the absorption mode would have to be adjusted to ensure that the mass-transfer front of the most volatile impurity does not endanger personnel.

Activated carbon outperformed polymeric resins and molecular sieves in a pressure-swing absorption system for regenerating air-purification media used to collect chemical agents (Stallings, 1984). Optimal performance was obtained at a purge-to-feed velocity ratio of 1.5 during 40-minute operation cycles. Zeolites outperformed activated carbon when pressure-swing absorption was used in the nonisothermal, adiabatic mode (Chue et al., 1995).

Pressure and temperature-swing absorption has been used for the removal of water that competes with toxic substances for the absorption sites on activated carbon (Coombes et al., 1994). In tests of the pressure-swing system, water from composite air-purification devices consisting of layered Amberlite XAD-4 resin and two commercial activated carbons (Chemviron BPL F3 and Sutcliff Speakman Type 607) was completely recovered. Each two-hour operating cycle consisted of four 30-minute steps:

- absorption at 10 bar and 75 liters per minute
- depressurization to ambient pressure while heating to 125°C with 5 liters per minute countercurrent flow
- cooling to ambient temperature with 10 liters per minute countercurrent flow
- repressurization with 20 liters per minute countercurrent flow

In this study, regeneration appears to have consumed 75 percent of the operation time and nearly half of the purified air.

Catalytic Oxidation

Catalytic oxidation is being developed as an advanced technology for NBC collective protection. Studies have focused on the feasibility of integrating catalytic oxidation/environmental control unit technology into a combat ground vehicle (Cag et al., 1995). Some of the elements of a protection system are: a catalytic reactor; a high-efficiency particulate air filter; an acid gas filter; a heater; volume, mass, and power requirements; cleaning and maintenance systems; waste disposal; and thermal signature.

Activated carbon as a filter for some acid gases (HBr, HF, NO and NO_2) has been evaluated previously (Buettner et al., 1988). Subsequent work with NO-NO_x and 3X catalysts showed that the majority of acid gases were condensed with the water in the environmental control unit, thereby minimizing the need for treatment of the effluent stream (Rossin, 1996). AS-1 and AS-2 NO_x absorbers developed by AlliedSignal's Aerospace Division have been shown to satisfy the post-treatment filter uptake, capacity, and durability requirements of the catalytic oxidation/environmental control unit system (Renneke, 1998).

FINDINGS AND RECOMMENDATIONS

Finding. Current challenges used to evaluate protective equipment do not reflect changes in threat levels.

Recommendation. The Department of Defense should reevaluate its requirements for materiel development to protect against liquid and vapor threats and revise design requirements, if appropriate.

Finding. PPE modules (e.g., masks, garments, gloves) were designed as independent items and then "retrofitted" to create an ensemble. They were also developed without adequate attention to various human factors issues, such as the integration of PPE with weapon systems.

Finding. The most serious risk from most CB agents appears to be from inhalation. Current doctrine allows for Mask-Only protection, but the mask seal could be broken while advancing from Mask-Only to MOPP 4 status.

Recommendation. A total systems analysis, including human factors engineering evaluations, should be part of the development process of the personal protective equipment system to ensure that the equipment can be used with weapon systems and other military equipment. These evaluations should include:

- the performance of individuals and units on different tasks in various realistic scenarios

- the interface of the mask and garments and potential leakage during an "advance" from Mask-Only to MOPP 4 status

Finding. Although researchers have good data from human factors testing that identifies serious performance (cognitive and physical) limitations as a result of wearing PPE, they have been unable to adequately relate these deficiencies to performance on the battlefield.

Recommendation. The Department of Defense should place greater emphasis on testing in macroenvironments and controlled field tests rather than relying mostly on systems evaluations for personal protective equipment.

Finding. Although the seal of the M40 mask is much improved over previous mask models, seal leakage continues to be a critical problem. The leakage can be attributed to (1) problems with the interface between the seal and the face, and (2) improper fit.

Recommendation. Additional research is needed on mask seals and mask fit. The research program should focus on seals, fit, and sealants (adhesives). The duration/severity of leaks, if any, during transitions in protective posture from one MOPP level to another should also be investigated. These data would be useful for future studies on long-term health effects of low-level exposures. In addition, training to fit masks properly should be conducted for all deployed forces equipped with mission-oriented protective posture equipment.

Finding. Although mask fit testing has been shown to improve protection factors 100-fold, the Air Force and Army have only recently begun deploying mask fit testing equipment and providing appropriate training protocols and supportive doctrine.

Recommendation. Doctrine, training, and equipment for mask fit testing should be incorporated into current joint service operations. The Department of Defense should deploy the M41 Mask Fit Test kit more widely.

Finding. Leakage around closures in personal protective equipment remains a problem.

Recommendation. The Department of Defense should continue to invest in research on new technologies to eliminate problems associated with leakage around closures. This research could include the development of a one-piece garment, the use of barrier creams on skin adjacent to closure areas, and other technologies still in the early stages of development.

Finding. Current gloves reduce tactile sensitivity and impair dexterity.

Recommendation. The Department of Defense should evaluate using a combination of barrier creams and lightweight gloves for protection in a chemical and/or biological environment. Multilaminate gloves should also be further explored.

Finding. An impermeable garment system is believed to provide the most comprehensive protection against CB agents. But impermeable barriers cause serious heat stress because they trap bodily moisture vapor inside the system. Permeable systems, which breathe and allow moisture vapor to escape, cannot fully protect against aerosol and liquid agents.

An incremental improvement could be achieved by using a semipermeable barrier backed with a sorptive layer. This system would allow the moisture vapor from the body to escape and air to penetrate to aid in cooling. The multilayer system would have some disadvantages, however. It would be bulky and heavy; and the sorptive layer is an interstitial space where biological agents could continue to grow because human sweat provides nutrients for growth of biological agents, which could prolong the period of active hazards. Countermeasures should be investigated to mitigate these problems.

Recommendation. The Department of Defense should investigate a selectively permeable barrier system that would be multifunctional, consisting of new, carbon-free barrier materials, a reactive system, and residual-protection indicators.

The carbon-free barrier materials could consist of: (1) smart gel coatings that would allow moisture/vapor transport and would swell up and close the interstices when in contact with liquid; (2) selectively permeable membranes that would allow moisture/vapor transport even in the presence of agents; (3) electrically polarizable materials whose permeability and repellence could be electronically controlled.

The reactive material could be smart, carbon-free clothing with gated membranes capable of self-decontamination. A reactive coating could also be applied to the skin in the form of a detoxifying agent (e.g., agent reactive dendrimers, enzymes, or catalysts capable of self-regeneration).

A residual-protection indicator would eliminate the premature disposal of serviceable garments and might also be able to identify the type of contamination. Conductive polymers could be used with fiber-optic sensors to construct the device.

Finding. Nanofiber technology is still in its infancy, and production capacity for nonfilter applications is not available in the United States or elsewhere.

Recommendation. The Department of Defense should evaluate the potential contributions of nanofiber technology to the development of personal protective equipment. An advanced protective garment should include nanofiber-impregnated yarn fabric or nanofiber/microfiber nonwoven fabrics.

Finding. The Department of Defense does not have enough collective protection units to meet the needs of deployed forces.

Recommendation. The Department of Defense should assess the needs of deployed forces for collective protection units in light of changing threats and the development of new personal protective equipment and provide adequate supplies of such equipment to deployed forces.

5

Decontamination

Decontamination is the process of removing or neutralizing chemical or biological agents so that they no longer pose a hazard. For military purposes, decontamination is undertaken to restore the combat effectiveness of equipment and personnel as rapidly as possible. Most current decontamination systems are labor and resource intensive, require excessive amounts of water, are corrosive and/or toxic, and are not considered environmentally safe. Current R&D is focused on developing decontamination systems that would overcome these limitations and effectively decontaminate a broad spectrum of CB agents from all surfaces and materials.

R&D on decontamination has evolved over the years. Ideally, these efforts would result in the identification and deployment of a "universal" decontaminating system. However, this has not happened. During and after the 1950s, most decontamination involved aqueous-based systems or the nonaqueous Decontamination Solution Number 2 (DS2), both of which have weaknesses. Aqueous-based systems require large amounts of water (often not available on a battlefield) and are very inefficient at removing agent that has been adsorbed onto or absorbed into a painted surface. In addition, the contaminated water must be gotten rid of. DS2 is too corrosive for many applications. Ongoing attempts to develop dry systems (referred to euphemistically as "magic pixie dusts") that would be easy to transport and use, would not require large amounts of fluids, and could replace DS2 or aqueous systems, have not yet been successful.

Based on the experiences of U.S. forces in the Gulf War and as a consequence of the breakup of the Soviet Union, the focus of the military has changed from defense against massive, large-area battlefield strikes against mobile forces to the defense of assets supporting force and power projection. Current U.S. military strategies are based on our ability to deploy forces rapidly to various theaters of operation (Joint Chiefs of Staff, 1996; Secretary of Defense, 1999).

Fixed sites that are critical to the deployment of troops have now become attractive and vulnerable targets for CB attack, increasing the importance of protecting them or, if protection is impossible, improving our ability to restore contaminated sites and equipment to operational status. The focus of R&D has, therefore, been shifted from the decontamination of mobile forces to the decontamination of fixed sites. The key differences between decontamination of fixed sites and mobile forces are summarized in Table 5-1.

The Joint Science and Technology Panel for CB Defense identified five functional areas where effective decontamination may be necessary in the event of a CB attack: (1) skin and personal equipment, (2) exterior equipment (field and fixed), (3) sensitive equipment, (4) interior equipment, and (5) large areas (land systems, seaport systems, ships at sea). Although these areas have some common needs, they also have significantly different vulnerabilities. Because the shortcomings of all current decontamination methods can be slightly mitigated but not eliminated through effective training, advances in technology will be necessary to increase the effectiveness of decontamination methods.

The skin decontamination technologies currently used make personnel more vulnerable to injury by increasing percutaneous absorption. It had been assumed that washing with either water or soap and water removes all contaminants. Experimental data, however, especially studies on humans with agricultural chemicals, have demonstrated that this is

TABLE 5-1 Differences between the Decontamination of Fixed Sites and Mobile Forces

Fixed Sites	Mobile Forces
• Power and water resources are readily available. • Transportation is not a key factor. • Personnel operating in contaminated environments may be subject to prolonged exposure. • Many items and many different materials must be decontaminated.	• Resources are limited and must frequently be transported in. • Assets must be transported. • During decontamination, personnel are subject to limited exposures from contaminated equipment in a relatively "clean" environment. • The number of items to be decontaminated is generally small.

not true. First, washing with soap and water does not remove all of the chemicals. Second, at certain times, bathing actually increases systemic penetration into the body (Wester and Maibach, 1999a). Because the decontamination of skin poses radically different challenges from the decontamination of personal equipment, the subject is addressed as a separate issue in the next section.

DECONTAMINATION OF SKIN

Risks and Challenges

The time between exposure of the skin and decontamination is critical. Ideally, decontamination should be done within the first two minutes, before the agent penetrates the skin, because topical decontaminants are not effective for chemical agents that have penetrated the skin (Hurst, 1997). However, decontamination after 15 minutes of exposure can still be of value although it may not be as effective.

Washing with soap and water has always been assumed to remove chemical and biological materials from the skin. However, recent evidence suggests that penetration and systemic absorption/toxicity may actually be increased by washing (Wester and Maibach, 1999b, 1999c). Washing is also ineffective for decontaminating painted surfaces. Appendix D describes *in vitro* and *in vivo* techniques for determining if skin has been decontaminated.

Mustard and other organophosphates do not cause any sensation as they pass through the skin. The person may not even know which areas of skin are contaminated. Thus, an individual may become aware of exposure only after considerable damage has been done. Because the speed of decontamination is critical, an indicator of exposure would be very useful. In fact, the rapidity of contamination removal is more important than the type of decontaminant.

The following problems are common to current and potential decontaminants: irritation of the skin, toxicity, ineffectiveness, and high cost. R&D to develop a skin decontaminant with the following traits is continuing (Chang, 1984; Hurst, 1997):

- capability of neutralizing chemical and biological agents
- safety (i.e., nontoxic and noncorrosive)
- easy application by hand
- ready availability
- rapid action
- no production of toxic end products

- stability in long-term storage
- short-term stability (i.e., after issue to the unit/individual)
- affordability
- no enhancement of percutaneous agent absorption
- nonirritating
- hypoallergenic
- easy disposal
- safe to the eyes

Technologies

In the 1970s, the U.S. Army developed the M258 skin decontamination kit, which was modeled on a Soviet kit recovered from Egyptian tanks during the Yom Kippur War. This kit consisted of two packets, one containing a towelette prewetted with phenol, ethanol, sodium hydroxide, ammonia, and water; and one containing a towelette impregnated with chloramine-B and a sealed glass ampoule filled with zinc chloride solution. The ampoule was broken and the towelette wetted with the solution immediately prior to use. Zinc chloride was used to maintain the pH of water between 5 and 6 in the presence of the chloramine-B, which would otherwise raise the pH to 9.5 (Leslie et al., 1991).

The M291 kit, a solid sorbant system for wiping bulk liquid agent from the skin, was adopted in 1989 and is currently in use (Yang et al., 1992; Yang, 1995). This kit is composed of nonwoven fiber pads filled with a resin mixture (trade name XE-555) developed by Rohm & Haas Company (Kerch, 1998). The resin is composed of an absorptive resin based on styrene/divinylbenzene, a high surface area carbonized macroreticular styrene/divinylbenzene resin, cation-exchange sites (sulfonic acid groups), and anion-exchange sites (tetraalkylammonium hydroxide groups) (Yang et al., 1992; Yang, 1995). The absorptive resin can absorb liquid agents, and the reactive resins promote hydrolysis reactions; however, in a recent study using nuclear magnetic resonance (NMR), neither VX nor a mustard simulant was hydrolyzed on the XE-555 resin surface during the first 10 days (Leslie et al., 1991). GD was slowly hydrolyzed with a half-life of about 30 hours. The effectiveness of the M291 kit depends primarily on the physical removal of the agent by wiping. The resin blend in the M291 kit was found to be less corrosive to the skin than the liquid in the M258 system.

Another decontamination kit, the M295, contains the same resin as the M291 and may be used to decontaminate personal equipment but not the skin. At present, the most universal chemical agent decontamination methods continue to be washing with water or water and soap, oxidation, and acid/alkaline hydrolysis (fresh 0.5 percent hypochlorite solution at an alkaline pH) (Ali et al., 1997; U.S. Army Medical Research Institute of Infectious Disease, 1998).

Because several biological agents pose a percutaneous threat to a contaminated individual, respiratory protection alone may not provide adequate protection, although in most instances respiratory protection will be sufficient for short-term protection, provided decontamination of the skin is initiated relatively quickly (Johnson, 1990; LeDuc, 1989; Mikolich and Boyce, 1990).

The 0.5 percent hypochlorite solution, which has been used since World War I, is currently recommended for decontamination of all biological agents (Ali et al., 1997). However, it cannot be used in abdominal wounds, open chest wounds, on nervous tissue, or in the eye.

Reactive Skin Decontaminant Lotion (RSDL), which was developed in Canada and is believed to contain phenoxides, oximates, a solvent (such as tetraglyme), and a thickener, is said to be effective for a number of chemical agents and some biological agents (Bannard et al., 1991).

The U.S. Army Medical Research Institute of Chemical Defense (USAMRICD) is developing a barrier cream based on perfluorocarbon formulations (Braue, 1998). The cream will be applied in a 0.15-mm thick layer and is expected to provide protection for six hours (four hours minimum) against liquid agents, including HD, lewisite, GD, and VX. The cream would lessen the need for immediate skin decontamination after exposure. The requirements for the cream include: no interference with other antidotes or pretreatments, no increase in vulnerability to detection, a minimum shelf life of three years, and catalytic reactivity. The extreme thickness of the cream layer is a serious limitation, however, because it interferes with the normal functioning of the skin.

Stoichiometric reagents in the cream would not be expected to decontaminate a significant quantity of agent. Therefore, attempts are being made to include reactive constituents in the formulation. Some reactive species under development are polyoxometalates, cross-linked enzyme crystals: organophosphorous hydrolase (OPH) and organophosphorous acid anhydrolase (OPAA), nanoscale metal oxides (magnesium oxide [MgO], calcium oxide [CaO], titanium oxide [TiO_2], manganese oxide [MnO_2]), polymer-coated metal alloys (titanium-iron-manganese, manganese-nickel, calcium-nickel), potassium persulfate ($K_2S_2O_8$), zero valence metals (iron/palladium, zinc/palladium), 2,3-butanedione monoxime (present in the Canadian RSDL), thermophylic bacterial enzymes, and benzoyl peroxide (Braue, 1998).

DECONTAMINATION OF EQUIPMENT, FACILITIES, AND LARGE AREAS

Risks and Challenges

The decontamination of equipment is complicated because different types of equipment must be decontaminated by different means. For example, personal equipment (e.g., rifles, tools, and other gear) must be decontaminated by a different process than sensitive equipment (e.g., communications equipment, navigational equipment, computers, and avionics), which, almost by definition, cannot be exposed to aqueous decontaminants or strong oxidizing or caustic solutions. Interior equipment (e.g., the interior of vehicles, aircraft, and shelters) have unique requirements because personnel are likely to operate in these confined areas with reduced protection. Exterior equipment and large areas, including pre-existing facilities, land and sea systems (e.g., roadbeds, airfields, buildings, seaports, and cargo loading docks), operationally fixed sites (e.g., command and control facilities and maintenance facilities), and transportable support structures (e.g., supply depots, medical facilities, and communications and intelligence collection facilities) have extensive surface areas that must be decontaminated. In addition, decontamination equipment for use in buildings must fit in a conventional elevator.

Technologies

Self-Decontaminating Materials and Protective Equipment

Self-decontaminating coatings, which could facilitate the rapid reuse of contaminated equipment, could be formulated with components capable of catalyzing the conventional hydrolysis and oxidation reactions of agents (Albizo et al., 1988; Medema et al., 1987). Examples include nanoclusters of semiconductors, zero-valent metals, functionalized polymers, and polyoxymetalates in polymers (Tadros, 1999). Other areas being researched include using solar radiation to activate decontaminating compounds and discarding contaminants by using strippable coatings. Although several options are in development, none of these techniques is ready to be used in the field. Some applications are summarized in Table 5-2.

Natural Decontamination (Water, Steam)

Probably the first (and most versatile) decontamination method is washing or spraying with water, water plus soap or detergent, or steam.

TABLE 5-2 Decontamination Coatings

Coating	Applicable Agents	Production State	Description
Chemical agent-resistant coating (CARC)	all	available	CARCs are polyurethane-based coatings designed to be chemically resistant to both chemical agents and decontaminants. When a chemical agent is deposited on the surface of a CARC coating, the surface repels the agent causing it to form droplets. The agent is then removed or decontaminated.
Sacrificial coatings	not specified	in development	Sacrificial coatings quickly absorb deposited chemical agents to reduce vapor hazards. Once the agent is absorbed into the sacrificial coating, the contaminated coating can either release itself from an uncontaminated substrate or it can be stripped off using relatively mild decontaminants, such as soapy water.
Self-decontaminating coatings	not specified	in development	Self-decontaminating coatings absorb deposited chemical agents to reduce vapor hazards. Once the agent is absorbed into the coating, active decontaminating agents can degrade or neutralize the agent.

Sources: Friel and Graham, 1989; Nene et al., 1988; Stevens and Henderson, 1987.

A serious drawback to this method is that, although most contaminants are removed and diluted, not all of them are neutralized or destroyed. To neutralize or destroy CB agents, bleach or other chemical reagents must be added; but the large volume of fluid used can cause logistics challenges, and contaminated runoff may cause environmental problems and require subsequent treatment.

Weathering (Natural Attenuation)

"Weathering" is a mode of decontamination in which natural sources of heat and ultraviolet radiation (sunlight), water (precipitation), and wind (evaporation and dilution) degrade contaminants on equipment, structures, and terrain. The effectiveness of weathering as a decontamination process depends on the persistence of the agent, as well as on meteorological and surface conditions. Some conditions that are favorable for decontamination by weathering (high wind or high temperature) can also spread contamination by resuspending contaminated particles or liquids in air or by volatilizing agents at high temperatures with no wind (producing a vapor hazard). Ordinarily, thickened agents are not effectively removed by weathering.

Standard Decontaminants (Bleach, Decontaminating Solutions)

In the 1950s, supertropical bleach (a mixture of 93 percent calcium hypochlorite and 7 percent sodium hydroxide) was standardized for use as a decontaminant because it is more stable in long-term storage and easier to spread than bleaching powder. Bleach reacts with mustard gas by oxidation of the sulfide to sulfoxide and sulfone and by dehydrochlorination to form nontoxic compounds, such as $O_2S(CHCH_2)_2$ (Price and Bullitt, 1943). The G-agents are converted by hydrolysis to the corresponding phosphonic acids because the hypochlorite anion behaves as a catalyst (Epstein et al., 1956). In acidic solution, VX is oxidized rapidly by bleach at the sulfur bond and dissolves by protonation at the nitrogen bond. At high pH values, however, the solubility of VX is significantly reduced, and the deprotonated nitrogen is oxidized leading to the consumption of greater than stoichiometric amounts of bleach (Yang et al., 1992; Yang, 1995). At high concentrations of about 5 percent, bleach has been shown to kill bacterial spores (Bloomfield and Arther, 1992; Sagripanti and Bonifacino, 1996; Williams and Russell, 1991).

DS2, introduced in 1960, is a nonaqueous liquid composed of 70 percent diethylenetriamine, 28 percent ethylene glycol monomethyl ether, and 2 percent sodium hydroxide (Beaudry et al., 1990; Richardson, 1972). The reactive component is the conjugate base $CH_3OCH_2CH_2O^-$. Although DS2 is a highly effective decontaminant for chemical agents, ethylene glycol monomethyl ether showed teratogenicity in mice, so replacement with propylene glycol monomethyl ether (DS2P) has been proposed (Talamo et al., 1994). DS2 attacks paints, plastics, and leather materials so contact time is limited to 30 minutes followed by rinsing with large amounts of water. Personnel handling DS2 are required to wear respirators with eye shields and chemically protective gloves. The reactions of

DS2 with mustard lead to elimination of hydrogen chloride. Nerve agents react with DS2 to form diesters, which further decompose to the corresponding phosphonic acids. DS2 is not very effective in killing spores. Only 1-log kill was observed for *Bacillus subtilis* after one hour of treatment (Tucker, 1998).

German C8, a microemulsion system developed in Germany, consists of 76 percent water, 15 percent tetrachloroethylene, 8 percent calcium hypochlorite, and 1 percent anionic surfactant mix (Ford and Newton, 1989). German C8 enhances the solubility of agents but contains chlorinated hydrocarbons that are environmentally persistent. It may also produce toxic by-products, such as vinyl chloride (a carcinogen).

Standard decontaminants are effective not only for chemical agents but also for most biological agents. Pathogens that form spores may be considered a special case because bacterial spores are highly resistant structures formed by certain gram-positive bacteria usually in response to stresses in their environment. The most important spore-formers are members of the *Bacillus* and *Clostridium* genera. Spores are considerably more complex than vegetative cells. The outer surface of a spore is the spore coat, typically a dense layer of insoluble proteins containing a large number of disulfide bonds. The cortex consists of peptidoglycan, a polymer primarily made up of highly cross-linked N-acetylglucosamine and N-acetylmuramic acid. The spore core contains normal (vegetative) cell structures, such as ribosomes and a nucleoid.

Many bacterial pathogens, some of which are biological warfare agents (e.g., *Bacillus anthracis*), protect themselves from hostile environments by forming spores. Considerable research has been carried out to investigate methods of killing or inactivating bacterial spores. Although spores are highly resistant to many common physical and chemical agents, a few antibacterial agents are also sporicidal. Because many powerful bactericides may only be inhibitory to spore germination or outgrowth (i.e., sporistatic) rather than sporicidal, they may postpone rather than eliminate a biological warfare threat (Tadros, 1999). Examples of sporicidal reagents (in high concentrations) are glutaraldehyde, formaldehyde, iodine and chlorine oxyacids, peroxy acids, and ethylene oxide. In general, these reagents are toxic and, therefore, of limited use for decontaminating personnel.

Nonstandard Decontaminants (Caustic Soda, Solvents)

The SBCCOM Edgewood Chemical Biological Center has developed a microemulsion system called the multipurpose chemical biological decontaminant. It consists of tetrachloroethylene, water, a high concentration of cationic surfactant, a cosurfactant (tetrabutyl ammonium hydroxide), Fichlor reagent (sodium dichloroisocyanurate), a hydrolysis catalyst (sodium 2-nitro-4-iodoxybenzoate [IBX]), and sodium borate (Walther and Thompson, 1988). The multipurpose decontaminant is more stable than the German C8 emulsion. Fichlor reagent acts by producing hypochlorous acid upon interaction with water.

Another product designed to eliminate the use of chlorinated solvent, called decontamination agent multipurpose (DAM), contains N-cyclohexyl-2-pyrolidone, calcium hypochlorite, and a surfactant mixture. Although multipurpose decontaminants look promising, none has been accepted as a completely effective substitute for DS2 (see the extensive bibliography in Day, 1996).

Trichlorotrifluoroethane FC-113 is electrically nonconductive, compatible with electronic components, and is currently used as a cleaning solvent. These properties suggested that it might be used to decontaminate military equipment. An exploratory Army study of FC-113 resulted in the development of a nonaqueous decontamination system that can be used for sensitive electronic equipment (e.g., night-vision goggles and communication equipment) (Richmond et al., 1990).

Reactions and Mechanisms

Reactions involved in detoxification of chemical agents may be divided into substitution and oxidation reactions.

Substitution Reactions

The rate of hydrolysis[1] of mustard and the nature of the products formed depends on the solubility of mustard in water and on the pH of the water. Mustard forms a cyclic sulfonium cation that reacts with nucleophilic reagents (Mikolajczyk, 1989; Yang et al., 1992; Yang, 1995). The dominant product is thiodiglycol, which may react with sulfonium ions to produce the secondary intermediates HD-TDG and CH-TDG (Figure 5-1).

The hydrolysis of sarin (GB) and soman (GD) occurs rapidly under alkaline conditions and produces the corresponding O-alkyl methylphosphonic acid. In contrast, the hydrolysis of VX with OH⁻ ions is more complex. In addition to displacement of the thioalkyl group, the O-ethyl group is displaced producing a toxic product known as EA-2192 (Yang et al., 1992, 1997; Yang, 1995).

---

[1]Hydrolysis is a chemical reaction in which a substance reacts with water, hydroxyl ions, or other nucleophiles and becomes a different substance.

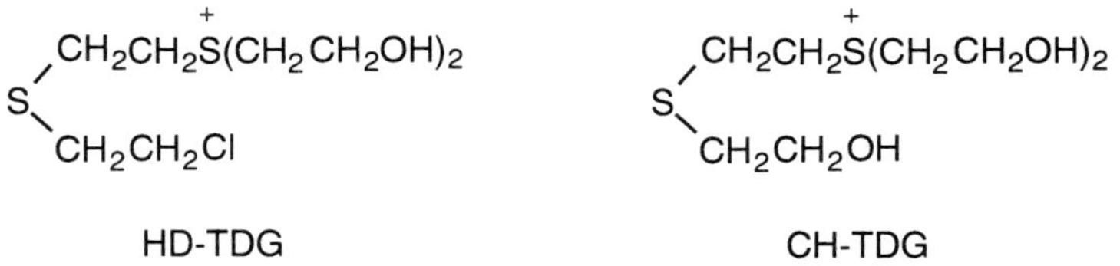

$$\text{S}\begin{smallmatrix}\nearrow \text{CH}_2\text{CH}_2\overset{+}{\text{S}}(\text{CH}_2\text{CH}_2\text{OH})_2 \\ \searrow \text{CH}_2\text{CH}_2\text{Cl}\end{smallmatrix} \qquad \text{S}\begin{smallmatrix}\nearrow \text{CH}_2\text{CH}_2\overset{+}{\text{S}}(\text{CH}_2\text{CH}_2\text{OH})_2 \\ \searrow \text{CH}_2\text{CH}_2\text{OH}\end{smallmatrix}$$

HD-TDG CH-TDG

FIGURE 5-1 Secondary products formed by hydrolysis of sulfur mustard.

Nucleophilic substitution at phosphorous centers involves addition to form a trigonal bipyramidal intermediate. Nucleophiles enter and depart the intermediate from an apical position. Electronegative groups, such as RO groups, preferentially occupy apical positions; groups that are bulky or π-electron donors, such as RS groups, occupy equatorial positions. If the lifetime of the TBP allows pseudorotation to occur, the final product will depend on the balance between apicophilicity and the tendency for the leaving group to disengage. The result is that P-S bond cleavage is favored over P-O bond cleavage by a factor of about five. Peroxyhydrolysis, however, using OOH$^-$ ions in alkaline medium was shown to involve quantitative P-S cleavage at rates 30–40 times the rate with OH$^-$. This selectivity was related to the relative base alkaline of the anionic nucleophile and the leaving anions (Yang et al., 1997).

Catalytic species (e.g., iodosobenzoate) have been used to accelerate substitution reactions. An example of the catalytic reactions of iodosobenzoate is shown in Figure 5-2 (Moss et al., 1983; Moss and Zhang, 1993). The compound was also functionalized to introduce surface activity and surfactant character to the active groups (Moss et al., 1986). Metal ion-amine complexes, with a surface active moiety, were also developed and shown to exhibit catalytic effects in substitution reactions (Courtney et al.,

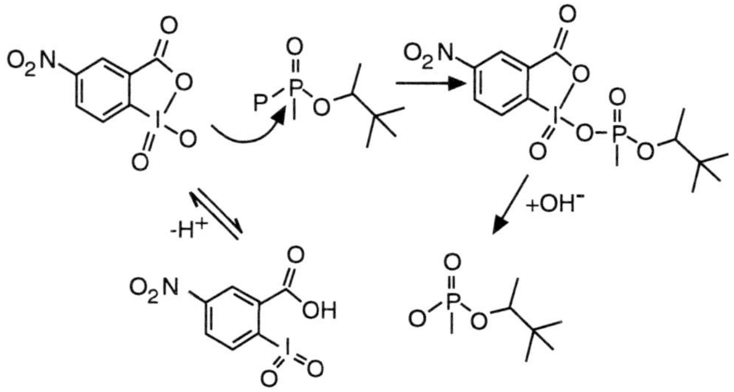

FIGURE 5-2 Catalytic acceleration of soman by iodobenzoate.

1957; Letts and Mackay, 1975; Menger et al., 1987). Enzymes, such as OPAA, have also been shown to accelerate substitution reactions with G and VX agents (Kolakowski et al., 1997; Ward, 1991).

Oxidation Reactions

Methods of oxidative decontamination are especially useful for mustard and VX (Yang et al., 1992; Yang, 1995) (see Table 5-3 for a list of oxidizing decontaminants and their characteristics). One of the first oxidants was potassium permanganate. Recently, oxone (a mixture of $KHSO_5$, $KHSO_4$, and K_2SO_4) has been developed. The reaction with VX in acidic oxone solutions is shown in Figure 5-3 (Mikolajczyk, 1989).

Several peroxy compounds have been shown to oxidize chemical agents (e.g., perborate, peracetic acid, m-chloroperoxybenzoic acid, magnesium monoperoxyphthalate, benzoyl peroxide, etc.). Recently, hydroperoxycarbonate anions produced by the reaction of bicarbonate ions with hydrogen peroxide, both relatively nontoxic compounds, have been shown to oxidize sulfur mustard and VX (Richardson et al., 1998; Tadros et al., 1998; Wagner and Yang, 1998). Polyoxymetalates are being developed as room-temperature catalysts for the oxidation of chemical agents, but the rates are reported to be slow at this stage of development (Rhule et al., 1998a, 1998b). Some of these compounds undergo a color change upon interaction with chemical agents (Kerch, 1998). This phenomenon is being exploited in formulations with barrier creams and solid sorbents to indicate the presence of chemical agents. Unfortunately, VX is often weaponized with a stabilizing agent, and under some conditions it can reform from decomposition products in the presence of that stabilizer. Thus, VX may reappear several hours after decontamination making decontamination less effective (McGuire et al., 1999).

Decontamination Media

The physical and chemical properties of agents must be taken into account for the design of an effective liquid decontaminant. Effective decontamination requires the rapid dissolution of agents in the decontamination medium. The hydrolysis of mustard, for example, shows that, at infinite dilution, the half-life for the hydrolysis reaction is four-and-a-half minutes; but for mustard in the form of 0.1-mm droplets, the half-life is six years (Harvey et al., 1997). For this reason, decontamination media based on nonaqueous, mixed solvent, emulsions, microemulsions, and self-organizing surfactant assemblies have been investigated. Agents are soluble in nonaqueous media, such as DS2, but they form large amounts of organic waste. Mixed solvent systems have better solubility, but

TABLE 5-3 Characteristics of Oxidizing Decontaminants

Decontaminant	Agents Decontaminated	State of Decontaminant
Sodium hypochlorite (bleach)	all	liquid
Calcium hypochlorite	G agents, VX, HD	liquid
High-test hypochlorite	GB, VX, HD	liquid
Dutch powder	GB, VX, HD	powder
Supertropical bleach	GB, VX, HD	liquid
Activated solution of hypochlorite	not specified	liquid
Fichlor	VX	liquid
Self-limiting activated solution of hypochlorite	not specified	liquid
Chloramine B	HD, VX	liquid
Chloramine T	G and H agents	liquid
Chlorine gas (Cl_2)	VX	gas
Potassium peroxy-monosulfate	VX, HD	liquid

Production Status	Description
available	Common household bleach
available	$Ca(OCl)_2$, a powerful oxidizing agent and an active component of both supertropical bleach and high-test hypochlorite. Hypochlorite ion (OCl^-) generated by an aqueous solution of $Ca(OCl)_2$
available	$Ca(OCl)Cl$ + calcium hypochlorite [$Ca(OCl)_2$] as a solid powder or a 7% aqueous slurry
in development	Bleach system composed of ($Ca(OCl)_2$ + MgO)
available	Combination of powerful oxidizers, calcium hypochlorite ($Ca(OCl)_2$), and a strong base (calcium oxide [CaO]); effective in the decontamination/detoxification of HD, G agents, and VX
available	Bleach system composed of 0.5% $Ca(OCl)_2$ + 1.0% sodium citrate + 0.2% citric acid + 0.05% detergent in water
available	Sodium dichloroisocyanurate ($C_3N_3O_3Cl_2Na$), a nitrogen-chloro oxidant that is commercially available; used in sanitizing, disinfecting, and bleaching agents in commercial bakeries and swimming pools
available	Bleach system composed of 0.5% $Ca(OCl)_2$ + 1.0% sodium citrate + 0.2% citric acid + 0.05% detergent in water
available	$C_6H_5ClNNaO_2S$, also known commercially as Neomagnol, an oxidant commonly used as an antibacterial agent; for decontaminating/detoxifying military chemical agents, chloramine-B is impregnated into a wetted towelette
available	Information not available
available	Cl_2, a very reactive gas that readily reacts with all elements except the rare gases and nitrogen; has been successfully used in the large-scale decontamination of VX
available	K_2O_4S, a component of oxone (a mixture of 2:1:1 [molar ratio] of $KHSO_5$:K_2SO_4:$KHSO_4$); in water, pH is 2.3 at 20°C; readily reacts with VX; The Lawrence Livermore National Laboratory has active decontamination program using this material

TABLE 5-3 Characteristics of Oxidizing Decontaminants (continued)

Decontaminant	Agents Decontaminated	State of Decontaminant
Ozone (O_3)	VX	gas
Sodium carbonate	not specified	liquid
BX24	not specified	liquid

Source: CBIAC, 1999.

oxidation and substitution reactions become slower as the polarity of the solvent decreases.

Cationic micellar solutions (Bunton et al., 1979, 1990; Bunton and Foroudian, 1993), vesicles (Jaeger et al., 1998; Schilling et al., 1997), and hydrotropes (Bunton and Quan, 1985; Tadros et al., 1986) (such as tetrapentyl ammonium bromide), and microemulsion systems (Bunton et al., 1983; Hermansky and Mackay, 1979; Menger and Elrington, 1991; Menger and Park, 1994) have all been shown to increase reaction rates with chemical agents (Figure 5-4).

All decontamination media require additives to reduce the viscosity of "thickened" agents. For example, monoethanolamine can be used to dissolve the common thickening agent n-methylpyrolidine.

Emerging Products

Enzymatic Decontaminants. Enzyme-based systems represent a new generation of CB agent decontaminants that are nontoxic, noncorrosive, environmentally safe, and light weight (LeJeune et al., 1998; LeJeune and

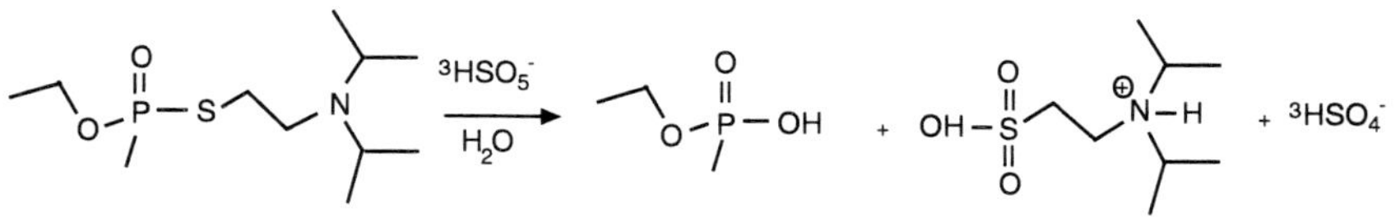

FIGURE 5-3 Oxidation of VX in acidic solution.

Production Status	Description
available	A reactive gas that can be used to react with and detoxify chemical agents; after detoxication, the space being detoxified can be vented
available	Information not available
in development	A powder that mixes easily with water and is commercially available; currently undergoing testing as an interim replacement for DS2

Russell, 1999; Russell and LeJeune, 1999). Enzymes are biological catalysts that significantly increase the rate of decontamination for specific chemical agents. Enzymatic decontaminants also have the potential for reducing logistical burdens because the materials can be shipped in dehydrated forms, and some enzyme systems can deactivate most G agents, as well as some V and H agents. The challenge is to develop an enzyme system that can decontaminate a broad spectrum of nerve and blister agents.

Challenges to producing adequate amounts of several of these enzymes have been overcome using molecular cloning and sequencing methods. Modern techniques for causing selective mutations and screening could reveal families of enzymes with broader applications.

The use of biological processes to destroy chemical warfare agents is at an early stage of development. Enzymes, such as OPH and OPAA,

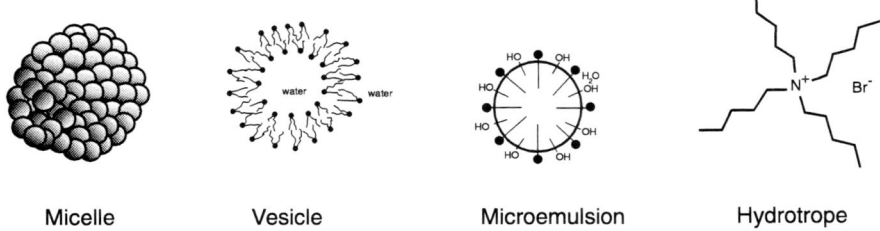

FIGURE 5-4 Molecular approaches to enhancing the solubility of chemical agents in liquid media.

have been shown to accelerate substitution reactions with G agents. Large-scale tests in fire-fighting solutions have demonstrated at least 99 percent destruction of GD in 15–30 minutes. Several V-agent enzyme systems have also been identified. Enzyme-compatible chemicals are being developed to enhance mustard hydrolysis (Kolakowski et al., 1997; Ward, 1991).

In general, enzyme systems have a number of attributes not common to conventional decontaminants (Table 5-4). Some of the disadvantages can be readily overcome. For example, enzymes are very specific with respect to the substrates on which they act. However, because they rarely interfere with each other's actions, mixtures of enzymes can be prepared that can attack several different agents. Several enzymes are currently available, and the methods for cloning the genes that produce them have been well established (Cheng et al., 1991; Lai et al., 1994). The cloned genes can be incorporated into various organisms (e.g., bacteria), which can then be cultured to produce large amounts of enzyme.

Several methods of developing enzymes with enhanced activity and/or the capability of deactivating multiple agents have been developed. These methods use directed mutations and rapid screening techniques to manipulate the genes that code for decontaminating enzymes (Longchamp, 1999). Maxygen, Inc., using Defense Advanced Research Projects Agency (DARPA) funding, is investigating the application of these methods to develop effective spore-degrading enzymes and to establish a collection of enzyme libraries for rapid screening against a wide variety of CB agents (Longchamp, 1999). Enzymes have also been incorporated into solid substrates, such as polymer foams. Polymer-bound enzymes may be more resistant to denaturation (e.g., by enzyme "folding"), a process in which distortion of the enzyme's molecular shape might alter the active site so that the substrate molecule could not bind effectively with the active site. The polymer incorporation technique may be compatible with the concept of "enzyme cocktails" that would take advantage of several different enzymes to combat several different agents with little cross-reactivity or interference. The polymer systems could be used as "wipes" or as sprayed powders. Polymer-stabilized enzymes could also be incorporated into detector systems.

The genes for several bacterial and squid enzymes have been cloned, sequenced, and expressed at high levels, which means that production of usable quantities of these enzymes could be feasible in the near term. OPH (bacterial V-agent enzyme) has been effective at reducing surface contamination by 99.9 percent; however, the contamination in the runoff was only degraded 12–40 percent after 20–40 minutes. G-agent enzymes removed 99.9 percent of GD from test plates with 99.8 percent degradation of the agent in runoff (Calomiris et al., 1994; Russell and LeJeune,

TABLE 5-4 Advantages and Disadvantages of Enzymatic Decontamination

Advantages	Disadvantages
Environmentally benign	High degree of specificity
High level of activity	Few enzymes currently available
Mild reaction conditions	Brief catalytic life
Minimal side reactions	Environmental sensitivity
Can be shipped in dry (lyophilized) form and reconstituted in the field	
Can use most freshwater or saltwater	

1999). These results appear to be quite promising. Enzyme preparations might also be used for decontamination of the skin.

Foam Decontaminants. Foam with enhanced physical stability for the rapid mitigation and decontamination of CB agents is being developed at Sandia National Laboratories (Tadros et al., 1998). The use of foam is attractive for the following reasons: (1) it requires minimal logistics support; (2) mitigation of agents can be accomplished in bulk, aerosol, and vapor phases; (3) it can be deployed rapidly; and (4) it has minimal runoff of fluids and no lasting environmental impact. The foam can be created and delivered by various methods. One preferred method is based on an aspiration, or Venturi, effect. The foam vehicle is sprayed under pressure through a restrictor, which causes a pressure drop that can draw air from the environment into the foam vehicle to create the foam. This method eliminates the need to pump additional air into a closed environment and minimizes the transport of agents to uncontaminated areas. This method also enhances the contact and mitigation of aerosols by formation of foam lamellae.

The effectiveness of foam decontaminants depends on the interaction of at least three factors: cationic surfactants (which enhance reaction rates with nucleophilic reagents), positively charged hydrotropes (which enhance the solubility and increase the reaction rates by providing a favorable molecular environment), and cationic polymers (which enhance compatibility reaction rates).

The additions of hydroperoxide and hydroperoxycarbonate ions (e.g., by adding hydrogen peroxide and sodium bicarbonate in alkaline medium) to the foam were found to enhance deactivation rates of both chemical and biological warfare agents. Synergistic effects were observed for the combined effects of the additives and the foam.

The decontamination of both real chemical warfare agents and biological warfare agent simulants by the combination of foam and additives has been demonstrated. Testing for chemical agents has been conducted with GD, VX, and HD. The half lives for the decontamination of these agents in the foam system is on the order of 2–10 minutes. Typical results with VX are shown in Figure 5-5 (Tadros et al., 1998). ^{31}P-NMR studies have shown exclusive cleavage of the P-S bond (see Figure 5-6). Results with *Bacillus subtilis* (Figure 5-7) show the synergistic effect of the foam and the oxidant. The realization that cleavage of a single bond eliminates toxicity in many chemical agents should be an area for further research. The target bonds can be attacked specifically and the rate and specificity can be conveniently monitored by NMR. However, with current equipment, reliable field units capable of NMR analysis are not practical.

The ability of the foam formulation to kill vegetative bacterial cells and viruses has also been demonstrated. Using the bacterium *Erwinia herbicola* as a biological simulant for vegetative cells, a 7-log kill in the foam within 15 minutes has been achieved.

However, this bacterium may not be a good simulant for the biological agents of concern. Complete deactivation was also achieved for the MS-2 bacteriophage (a simulant for biological agent viruses) in 30 minutes.

Gel Decontaminants. Lawrence Livermore National Laboratory is developing an aqueous gel containing the oxidation reagent peroxymonosulfate (oxone) in acidic medium. The gel is formed from fumed amorphous

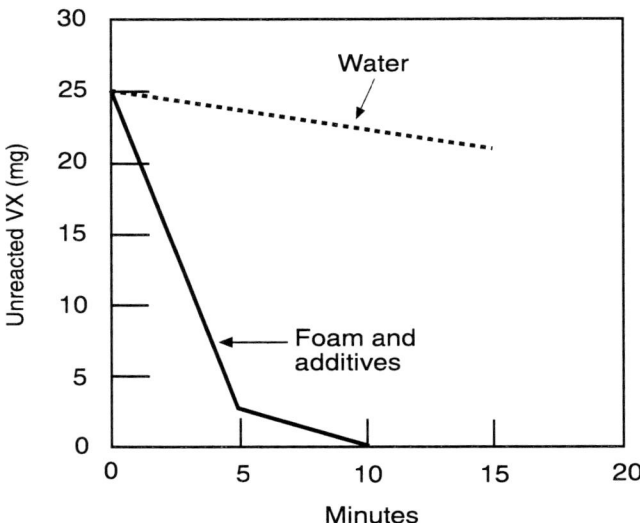

FIGURE 5-5 Decontamination of paper treated with 25 mg VX per 25 cm^2.

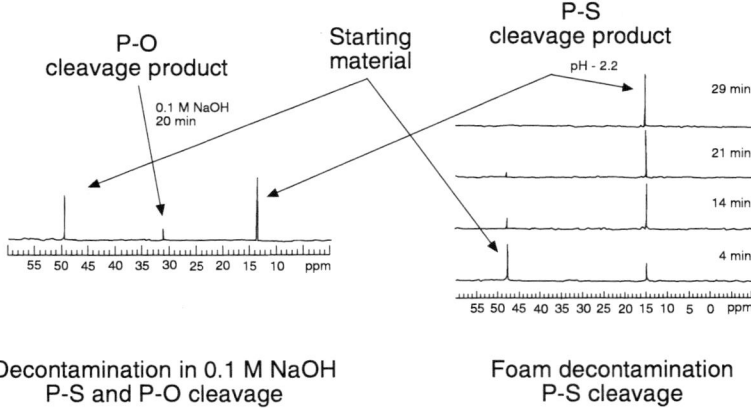

FIGURE 5-6 ^{31}P NMR study of the decontamination of O-ethyl-S-ethyl phenyl phosphonothioate.

silica particles, which can efficiently catalyze the hydrolysis of P bonds in G agents. The gel is thixotropic in nature, and the viscosity can be varied allowing the material to "stick." The gel has been tested on a variety of different materials using surrogates, and testing with actual agents is under way (Raber et al., 1998). The material residue has been shown to be environmentally acceptable.

The gel is sprayed on, allowed to dry, and then vacuumed up. The gel can attach to vertical and inverse surfaces. In a test with concrete and asphalt contaminated with VX and GD, an analysis after treatment showed that more than 97 percent of the cholinesterase-inhibiting capability had been destroyed. When HD was tested, residual activity was reduced to nondetectable levels. Some tests have been less successful, however. For example, GD was effectively removed from carpet but was less effectively removed from painted surfaces. The gel has also been tested against BG spores and found to reduce the number of spores by "6 logs" (i.e., no spores were detected after treatment).

Tri-n-butyl Phosphate (BCTP) Emulsion. Researchers at the University of Michigan and Novavax, Inc., have developed an antimicrobial emulsion with low toxicity consisting of soybean oil, Triton X-100, water, and a solvent (tri-n-butyl phosphate, known as BCTP). This material was shown to kill anthrax spores both in a culture dish and in mice exposed to anthrax through a skin incision. The authors claim that BCTP causes the spores to revert to an active bacterial state. In four to five hours, the spore

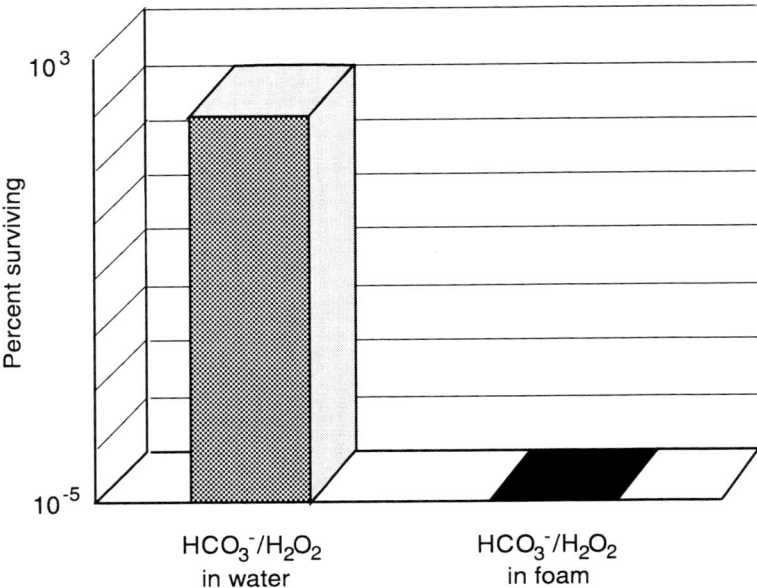

FIGURE 5-7 Foam decontamination of *Bacillus subtilis* spores after one hour of treatment. Demonstration of synergistic effects of the mild oxidant and the foam.

outer membrane changes, allowing the solvent to strip away the exterior membrane. The detergent then degrades the spore interior. A "1-log" kill (i.e., reduction in activity by a factor of 10) was reported during this time period (Reuter, 1998).

Gaseous Decontamination

Gases. Gas-phase reagents would be attractive for decontamination if the decontaminating gas is environmentally acceptable. The advantage of gas decontamination is that gases can penetrate (diffuse) and could be used to complement other decontamination techniques. Ozone, chlorine dioxide, ethylene oxide, and paraformaldehyde have all been investigated as decontaminants. All of these are known to be effective against biological agents. Reports by SBCCOM have shown that ozone is not effective as a decontaminant for GD (Bartram et al., 1998). Ozonic decontamination of VX leads to cleavage of the P-O bond and the formation of toxic products (Bartram et al., 1998). However, the effectiveness of ozone for killing spores in a high-humidity environment has been well established (Currier, 1999).

Vapor of hydrogen peroxide (VHP) is now used commercially for sterilization, and the sporicidal effects of VHP have been reported. A significant advantage of VHP is that it breaks down through a simple catalytic process into water vapor and oxygen, eliminating the emission of any dangerous by-products. Sandia National Laboratories is considering the development of a mixture of hydrogen peroxide (H_2O_2), carbon dioxide (CO_2), and water vapors to produce the active species hydroperoxycarbonate *in situ*.

Reactive Plasma. Los Alamos National Laboratories has developed an atmospheric-pressure plasma source to generate chemically reactive effluent for neutralizing chemical and biological agents (Selwyn and Currier, 1999). This approach is "dry," requires no subsequent cleanup or waste disposal, and can potentially decontaminate surfaces and equipment. The system could be modified to produce reactive metastables and/or radicals that may kill bacteria and viruses used as biological agents and might also be used to neutralize chemical agents.

The method is based on the development of a small electrical discharge in the space between two opposing insulated flat-plate electrodes connected to a high-voltage source at alternating radio frequencies. A large number of short-lived but high instantaneous current microdischarges are uniformly distributed over the discharge space. Energetic electrons are produced that lead to the creation of free radicals in the gas flowing between the electrodes. Because of the short duration of the microdischarges and low ion mobilities, the electrical energy is primarily coupled into electron channels so that the electrons, ions, and gas molecules do not equilibrate. Thus, the electrons are "hot," and the other species are "cold." This results in a very efficient transfer of electrical energy to electronic excitation of molecules and chemical processes at essentially ambient temperatures and pressures. One could actually expose skin or other heat-sensitive surfaces to such plasmas without being burned.

Innovatek, Inc., is commercializing a hand-held, low-power, corona discharge plasma flare that operates at atmospheric pressure and low temperatures for surface sterilization (Irving, 1998). In laboratory testing, the device demonstrated high-efficiency destruction of *Bacillus subtilis* and DMMP.

Reactive plasma units might also be used to monitor chemical agents. By analyzing the absorption bands in the plasma discharge, the presence of chemical agents can be detected. Thus, this technique has the potential of providing simultaneous decontamination and detection.

Technology in this area is developing rapidly. Current innovations include:

- plasma/peroxide systems for the decontamination of biological warfare agents
- plasma "blankets" that run at 30W and can be wrapped around small objects, such as a rifle
- plasma air purifiers that could augment or replace conventional filters

There may be problems with scale (i.e., producing enough plasma to cover a large area), but for decontamination or sterilization of delicate surfaces on objects the size of soldiers, electronics, or optics, these techniques are exciting. Because of their speed, low power requirements, and lack of residual products, this technology may be the method of choice for the decontamination of sensitive surfaces.

Supercritical Fluids. SBCCOM has initiated a program to extract chemical agents from contaminated sensitive equipment using supercritical carbon dioxide (Joint Science and Technology Panel for CB Defense, 1999). Supercritical fluids exhibit very high mass-transfer rates because of their liquid-like density, gas-like viscosity, and negligible surface tension. Carbon dioxide was selected because it is nontoxic, nonflammable, inexpensive, has a low supercritical temperature (31°C), and has high compressibility. In addition, no water, heat, or radiation (which could affect sensitive equipment) would be required.

A combination of extraction and simultaneous decontamination with reagents soluble in carbon dioxide has also been considered. Problems that must be solved before this technology could be used include the placement of equipment into reactor vessels and the need to transport and handle tanks of liquid carbon dioxide.

Radiation, Pressure, and other Techniques

Ultraviolet Activated Oxidation Systems. The photolysis of hydrogen peroxide, ozone, and other oxidants by ultraviolet radiation generates highly reactive intermediates, such as hydroxyl radicals, that can then degrade agents (Bolton and Stevens, 1995). These processes are called advanced oxidation processes. Ferrioxalate anions were found to absorb both in the ultraviolet and near-visible region at 500 nm yielding hydroxyl radicals. This method has the potential of using solar light as the energy source.

Ionizing Radiation. Ionizing radiation can include x-rays, gamma rays, high-intensity ultraviolet rays, and electron beams. Experimental measurements, presented as D_{10} values (i.e., the dose level required to reduce the sample population by a factor of 10), have been made of the effects of radiation on spores and bacteria. Typical D_{10} values for a number of spores and bacteria are 100–300 Krad (Ito et al., 1993). A minimum of $3D_{10}$ is required, and a level of $6D_{10}$ is considered a sterilization level. Thus, the dose required for typical spore agents ranges from 1 to 3 Mrad. Limited data are available on the effects of radiation on chemical agents and biological toxins. The D_{10} values for other organic molecules range from 0.3 to 5.0 Mrad (Gray and Hilarides, 1995; Turman et al., 1998).

An interesting application of radiation for decontamination would involve the use of electron beams (McKnight et al., 1999). The main components of the system would include some type of electron "gun," an accelerator, a power conditioning and control system, and shielding. In the field, shielding could be provided by soil so that bulky shielding material would not have to be transported. Large objects and runoff water are potential decontamination targets for electron beams.

Ionizing radiation is routinely recommended for the sterilization of prepackaged medical devices, and a 2,500-rad dose is generally effective for sterilization. Microorganisms are inactivated by the radiation that attacks water molecules within the organism creating intermediate hydrolysis products that result in complete inactivation. Because the radiation dose can be calculated with great reliability, the process is highly predictable.

The high penetration range of ionizing radiation (i.e., ability to penetrate beyond walls, cracks, ducting, etc.) makes it suitable for the decontamination of large areas, such as fixed sites. The major hazards associated with this technology are high voltage and radiation, both of which can be potentially mitigated. No residual waste or radioactivity is left behind after treatment provided that the energy of the exciting beam does not exceed about 10 million electron volts (MeV) (Battelle Memorial Institute and Charles Williams, Inc., 1999).

Several applications for decontamination by ionizing radiation have been considered (Irving et al., 1997). High-energy radiation could provide a method for destroying agent while it is still inside a bomb-type canister, which would be an effective way of dealing with terrorist threats of most biological agents and some chemical agents. Radiation might also be used to decontaminate large areas, such as airstrips, highways, and seaports. The kill rate increases logarithmically with time, so the percentages of decontamination would increase as the time of irradiation increased.

Operationalizing radiation methods will require the detection of chemical warfare missiles and the availability of compact beam accelerators. Several accelerator technologies could be used (Turman et al., 1998); and several low-power options are already commercially available. The

Titan Beta Linac produces a beam of 10 MeV at a maximum power of 15 kW; the beam can be extracted through a thin metal foil for propagation through the atmosphere for a short range. The beam is scanned in one dimension over a distance of about 100 cm at the exit window. A similar system has been fielded on a truck bed for mine detection applications (Figure 5-8). Other systems are the Canadian AECL (radio-frequency accelerator with 9.5 MeV 50kW beam output) and the Belgium Rhodatron accelerator (10 MeV, 150 kW). High-current, high-power beams can be produced with linear inductive voltage-adder accelerators, such as the RHEPP II accelerator at Sandia National Laboratories that produces a 2.5 MeV, 20 kA, 3 KJ pulsed beam. This technology has the potential to produce beam power with an average of 300 kW at a repetitive rate of 100Hz. With some miniaturization of the superconducting elements, conventional radio-frequency accelerators could fit on a truck bed.

Feasibility studies are being conducted at Sandia National Laboratories to validate the concept that electromagnetically induced alteration of tertiary molecular structure is sufficient to deactivate biological agents. The wavelength will be selected based on absorption characteristics of the agents in the microwave region. The system would be fast and energy efficient and could be used on the surfaces of sensitive equipment (Tadros, 1999).

CURRENT DOCTRINE AND TRAINING

Army Field Manual (FM) 3-5/Fleet Marine Force Manual 11-10 (U.S. Army and U.S. Marine Corps, 1993) provides detailed guidelines for

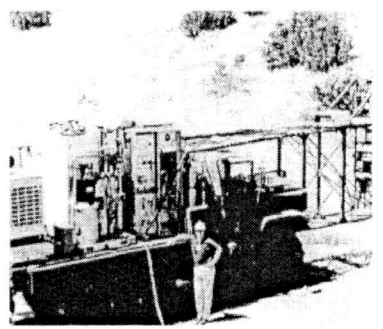
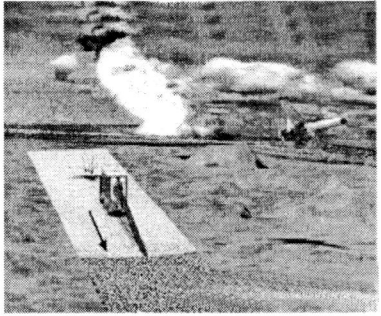

a. b.

FIGURE 5-8 (a) High-energy accelerator fitted on a truck. (b) Large-area decontamination with ionizing radiation.

decontamination operations. One of the basic messages of this doctrine is that decontamination is costly in terms of manpower, time, space, and materiel; the same resources required to fight the battle.

Therefore, commanders must use them wisely to sustain combat operations. To limit the spread of contamination, commanders are advised to decontaminate equipment and personnel as soon and as far forward as possible, decontaminating only as much equipment and as many personnel as necessary. Commanders are also advised to decontaminate chemical agents first because decontamination methods for chemical agents are also believed to be effective for neutralizing or removing biological contamination, but not vice versa.

Decontamination is only briefly mentioned in *Joint Doctrine for Nuclear, Biological and Chemical Defense* (Joint Chiefs of Staff, 1995). This document does not include detailed operational guidelines but does iterate the concepts spelled out in *FM 3-5/FMFM 11-10* (U.S. Army and U.S. Marine Corps, 1993). It also suggests that, depending on the CB agent, decontamination may not be necessary because of natural weathering effects. Natural decontamination by weathering, ultraviolet, and thermal processes has been effectively used as a basis for Air Force procedures for spot decontamination in selected areas.

Army doctrine related to training in decontamination states that all individuals will be trained in basic decontamination skills using individual and unit decontamination equipment and that leaders will ensure that their units are proficient in decontamination procedures (U.S. Army and U.S. Marine Corps, 1993). Joint doctrine does not specifically mention training in decontamination (Joint Chiefs of Staff, 1995) except that each service will incorporate NBC defense training into its overall training plan for units and individuals. The degree to which training is effective and/or being provided is not known because DoD does not have a mechanism for assessing the status of training (DoD, 1999).

The shift in military strategy in the 1980s to dependence on force projection capabilities has resulted in profound changes in attitude toward decontamination. Several areas of potential vulnerability were identified in a computer simulation (called CB 2010) of a covert CB attack on forces during the process of deployment from the continental United States (CONUS) to the Middle East (Booz-Allen and Hamilton, 1997).

The simulation showed that CONUS ports of embarkation were vulnerable and that CB attacks could delay deployment and degrade the effectiveness of fighting forces. In this scenario, the mission was seriously compromised, and some military objectives were not achieved. The purpose of the CB attack was not necessarily to kill, but to disrupt and delay deployment.

In a more recent deployment exercise at Pope Air Force Base and Fort Bragg, the computer scenario was incorporated into a war game (Raines, 1999). In a covert CB attack, simulated thickened mustard was dropped from two crop-duster aircraft. The attack targeted key deployment areas and mission-critical assets. The following lessons were learned:

- The attack successfully delayed and disrupted deployment. The delay, which was longer than one day, was significantly longer than was predicted by CB 2010.
- No DoD guidelines address CB threats against military operations in CONUS.
- No monitoring capability or chemical protective equipment was available for the deploying troops because their gear had been packed for transport.
- Post-attack detection and decontamination facilities and equipment were also packed, which delayed decontamination.
- No decontamination standards were available for certifying that contaminated equipment could be returned to operational status.
- Nondeploying (or nonmobility) personnel did not have equipment and had not been trained in CB defense.
- The medical facilities were overwhelmed by the casualties and were not prepared to treat contaminated personnel.

This exercise clearly identified discontinuities between doctrine and training. At the very least, facilities and equipment that are critical to a force deployment mission should be identified and appropriate plans developed to protect and/or decontaminate critical assets. Guidelines for responding to a CB attack in CONUS are clearly necessary.

The relationship between doctrine (or guidance) and risk with respect to decontamination is complicated, especially because the risk has not been quantified. USACHPPM has drafted *Short-Term Chemical Exposure Guidelines for Deployed Personnel*, which provides exposure guidelines that could be used "as criteria to identify potential risks that should be considered in deployment mission decision-making and overall risk management" (U.S. Army CHPPM, 1999, p. 1-2). These guidelines, which were intended for use during deployments and exercises outside CONUS, were not intended to be used as mandatory exposure standards.

The key question in the development of doctrine on decontamination is long-term exposure to low-level concentrations in a contaminated environment. The doctrine would have to establish the sufficient level of decontamination (i.e., "how clean is clean enough?"). Setting of exposure guidelines is a critical step in the assessment of risk and provides a basis for managing the risk (which relates to doctrine).

The severity and extent of the effects of exposure to CB agents depends on the following factors:

- individual sensitivity
- duration of the exposure
- agent concentration
- aggravating or mitigating conditions (i.e., medical pretreatments, health status, other chemicals, etc.)

USACHPPM has proposed 1-day and 14-day military air guideline (MAG) levels (exposures for 24 hours/day for 1 or 14 days). These levels may appear to be conservative when compared to the Occupational Safety and Health Administration (OSHA) standards or other industrial hygiene guidelines. However, USACHPPM assumes exposures of 24 hours/day while industrial guidelines are based on 8 hour/day exposures.

Field commanders are responsible for deciding what risks are necessary for accomplishing their missions. Making informed decisions and managing the overall risks in the deployment environment require information on agent concentrations. The MAGs for chemical warfare agents listed in Table 5-5 are for concentrations that produce minimal and severe effects after 1-day and 14-day exposures.

Relating doctrine to risk in the area of decontamination will first require establishing guidelines for what constitutes acceptable risk and then

TABLE 5-5 Military Air Guidelines for Chemical Warfare Agents

Agent	1-hour MAGs (ppm)		Time-Weighted Average of 1-day to 14-day MAGs (ppm)
	Minimal Effects	Severe Effects	
Tabun	0.008	0.10	0.000010
Sarin	0.008	0.10	0.000010
Soman	0.003	0.05	0.000003
VX	0.0015	0.02	0.000030
Sulfur mustard	0.05	no data	0.003[a]
Phosgene	0.10	1.00	0.01

[a]Not to exceed at any time.

Source: U.S. Army CHPPM, 1999.

developing the doctrine and training protocols for limiting exposure. At the present time, some of the elements necessary for developing doctrine are inadequate. For example, detection capabilities are not designed for the decontamination environment. The current fast-response methods are not sensitive enough, and the sensitive, definitive assays are very time consuming and not easily adaptable for field use. If the MAGs were accepted as guidelines for managing risks, estimates of exceedances could be made (i.e., an "effects-based" decontamination goal). If an effects-based goal cannot be established, the lower limit of detectability by the most sensitive method available could be adopted as the decontamination goal by default (i.e., an "analysis-based" decontamination goal).

Because doctrine is not strongly related to risk, several serious problems remain all but unsolvable. First, no standards can be established for returning previously contaminated equipment to service. Second, decontamination doctrine is not consistent across services. And third, problems are more complicated when joint forces or coalition forces are involved.

FINDINGS AND RECOMMENDATIONS

As belief in the CB threat has increased, decontamination has received more attention, but few changes in funding have resulted. No extensive, planned, organized research programs are being conducted, and many issues remain unresolved.

Finding. Just as only a few benchmarks for the removal of MOPP gear have been established (because detection technology is inadequate), few benchmarks of decontamination levels have been established. Therefore, it is difficult to know when it is safe to return equipment to operational status and impossible to "certify" that previously contaminated equipment can be transported to a new location, especially a location in the United States.

Recommendation. The Department of Defense should initiate a joint service, interagency, international cooperative effort to establish decontamination standards. Standards should be based on the best science available and may require the development of new models for setting benchmarks, especially for highly toxic or pathogenic agents.

If residual decontamination levels are based on ultraconservative toxicity and morbidity estimates, returning contaminated equipment becomes impractical. Benchmarks for decontamination should be based on highly accurate, reliable, up-to-date toxicity data.

Finding. Although significant progress is being made with limited resources in exploring decontamination technologies that may be effective, no organized, integrated research program has been developed to meet the new challenges and objectives that have been posed (i.e., environmentally acceptable decontamination). Various agencies are actively pursuing many projects, but they are not well coordinated and do not have clear priorities for fixed-site programs, casualty management, and sensitive equipment programs.

Recommendation. The Department of Defense (DoD) should coordinate and prioritize the chemical/biological research and development (R&D) defense program, focusing on the protection of deployed forces and the development of environmentally acceptable decontamination methods. DoD should also establish the relative R&D priority of decontamination in the chemical/biological defense program.

Finding. Recent developments in catalytic/oxidative decontamination (enzymes, gels, foams and nanoparticles) appear promising for decontaminating a wide range of CB agents.

Recommendation. Research on enzyme systems for battlefield decontamination (especially for small forces) should be given high priority because they could be used to decontaminate both personnel and equipment and would not require large volumes of water or complicated equipment.

Recommendation. The Department of Defense should continue to develop other catalytic/oxidative systems for larger scale decontamination. If possible, these systems should be less corrosive and more environmentally acceptable than current methods.

Finding. Low-power plasma technology has been shown to be effective for decontaminating sensitive equipment and has the potential of incorporating contaminant-sensing capabilities.

Recommendation. The Department of Defense should continue to develop plasma technology and other radiation methods for decontaminating equipment.

6

Testing and Evaluation

The testing and evaluation of equipment, methodologies, and toxicological factors are critical for the development of CB defensive strategies. Testing must be done on several different levels, ranging from rigorous tests of components of protective equipment to assessments of current doctrine and training by means of simulations and exercises (including war games).

TOXICOLOGICAL TESTING

In keeping with the principles and spirit of the nonproliferation agreements entered into by the United States, U.S. policy prohibits most tests using real agents and studies with human volunteers (except with surrogate agents). Therefore, most human and animal studies are done with simulants, which may not be adequate surrogates for potential threat agents (Rhodes et al., 1998). In fact, the airborne behavior of simulants and real agents differ significantly, as do their dermal penetration and metabolic effects. These differences make estimating absorbed doses and toxic effects extremely difficult. Thus, based on simulant challenge data, it is extremely difficult to determine whether specific pieces of equipment meet requirements.

Although fewer studies have been done on dermal penetration than on the inhalation or ingestion of agents, the current clothing R&D program is predicated on the need to avoid a percutaneous challenge from agents. Current efforts to develop a new protective ensemble (i.e., JSLIST) and chemically protective undergarments are based on the principle of preventing CB agents from contacting the skin. Although dermal contact is an obvious danger for blister-type agents, such as nitrogen and sulfur mustards, the percutaneous threat of other agents (e.g., G or V agents or biological agents) has not been established. The available data on percutaneous absorption and the physiological effects of agents absorbed percutaneously are very limited.

For the most part, percutaneous threats from chemical agents have been defined using data from animal studies. Percutaneous threats from biological agents have been defined mostly anecdotally; however, there are situations in which skin contact with biological agents has been shown to have adverse effects (Johnson, 1990; LeDuc, 1989; Mikolich and Boyce, 1990). Because the requirements for protection against percutaneous threats are based on such sketchy data, the goals, requirements, and results of the R&D programs are necessarily based on uncertainties. Strategies for rigorous testing of dermatological exposures will be necessary in two important areas: (1) quantifying skin uptake and resultant toxicology, and (2) determining the efficacy of skin decontamination.

Tests of percutaneous toxicology can be interpreted using well defined models. DPK models are based on relationships among the amount of agent presented to the skin surface, the amount of drug (or toxic chemical) absorbed into the body, and the rate of contamination. Dermatopharmacodynamic (DPD) models determine the CB effects of the absorbed dose (Gupta et al., 1993; Marzulli and Maibach, 1991; Zhai and Maibach, 1996). DPK models describe agent uptake as a function of dose and time; while, DPD models are used to evaluate the relationship between the concentration at the effector or target site and the biologic effect. DPK models may provide kinetic details and suggest mechanisms that could supplement traditional clinical studies. Therefore, DPK models can be used to evaluate both percutaneous absorption (Gupta et al., 1993; Shah et al., 1991, 1993; Zhai and Maibach, 1996) and dermal decontamination (Wester and Maibach, 1999b).

Evaluation of Percutaneous Penetration

DPD models have been used to ascertain bioavailability from percutaneous exposure. Bioavailability can be defined as the rate and extent to which the administered toxic agent is absorbed via the skin and becomes available at the site of chemical action and/or reaches the general circulation. Thus, the approach based on these models can be used to evaluate the absorption and toxicity of agents during dermal exposures, the effectiveness of decontamination, and the degree of protection provided by protective treatments, such as applications of barrier creams.

DPD models can be used to estimate the movement of chemicals into the first organ system (skin), and quantities can be determined indirectly by noninvasive bioengineering techniques (e.g., colorimetry, transepidermal water loss, laser doppler velocimetry, etc.) (Berardesca et al., 1995a, 1995b; Elsner et al., 1994; Frosch et al., 1993a; McDougal, 1991, 1998; Wester and Maibach, 1999c; Wilhelm et al., 1997).

The following 10 factors should be included in rigorous evaluations of percutaneous absorption (Wester and Maibach, 1983):

- vehicle release
- absorption kinetics
- excretion kinetics
- cellular and tissue distribution
- substantivity
- wash and rub resistance
- volatility
- binding
- anatomical pathways
- cutaneous metabolism

For more detailed scientific information on these 10 factors, see Appendix E.

Vehicle Release

Percutaneous absorption of a drug from a vehicle (i.e., mechanism of transport) depends on the partition of the chemical between the vehicle and the skin and the solubility of the drug in the vehicle (e.g., isopropyl alcohol, dimethyl sulfoxide). Solubility, concentration, and pH of the drug can influence interactions among the vehicle, the active chemical, and the skin. Vehicles sometimes contain agents, such as urea, that can enhance percutaneous absorption. In some cases, the vehicle itself may enhance absorption or change skin integrity. An occlusive vehicle, for example, could alter skin hydration.

Absorption Kinetics

Absorption kinetics vary according to a number of factors: (1) skin application site, (2) individual variations, (3) skin condition, (4) occlusion, (5) chemical concentration and surface area, and (6) number of applications. Percutaneous absorption in humans and animals varies with the anatomical site to which the compound is applied. Even if application conditions remain the same (e.g., application site, compound, concentration, dose, vehicle), absorption can vary by several-fold because of individual variations.

Any change in skin condition, especially changes in the barrier function of the stratum corneum, whether natural or inflicted, may alter percutaneous absorption. Skin condition also changes with age; the stratum corneum of preterm infants is not fully developed and, therefore, is more permeable than in a fully developed infant. Damage, disease, and occlusion (overhydration) may also increase absorption levels. Percutaneous absorption is often increased when the application site is occluded. Chemical concentration and surface area are also critical parameters in determining the amount of absorption. As the concentration of the applied dose increases, the total amount absorbed increases. As the surface area of the applied dose increases, the total amount of absorption also increases.

If any topically administered compound is applied more than once a day, the topical exposure may be chronic. Absorption from one application of a high concentration may be greater than the same concentration applied in equally divided doses. The mechanisms controlling this are not yet understood.

Excretion Kinetics

A potentially toxic chemical will be more or less damaging depending on the rate of excretion or retention in the body. For instance, although lindane and hexachlorophene are not well absorbed, their potential for toxicity is enhanced by their slow excretion and storage in lipid compartments. In general, water-soluble compounds are rapidly excreted and are generally less toxic.

Cellular and Tissue Distribution

The concentration of chemical in the skin is usually highest near the surface and lowest in the dermis. Differences in percutaneous absorption depend not only on the thickness, surface area, and number of cell layers in the stratum corneum, but also on lipid composition and concentration distribution of the chemical in the skin layers.

Substantivity

Substantivity is a measure of the portion of the applied dose that binds to the skin surface and may eventually be lost by skin exfoliation. When radioisotopes are used, substantivity can be monitored by surface counting; otherwise, skin stripping cellophane tape can be used.

Wash and Rub Resistance

A compound applied to skin surface can be partially removed by washing or rubbing. Mechanical stress on the skin, such as friction from clothing, may alter both the distribution of the applied dose and percutaneous absorption.

Volatility

Volatility refers to the partition of a chemical between its vehicle on the skin surface and the surrounding air (an important factor for mosquito repellents). Accurate determinations of percutaneous absorption *in vitro* or *in vivo* with animal and human models require simulations of air flow with volatile chemicals.

Binding

Chemicals may bind to the stratum corneum (i.e., substantivity) or to other tissue compartments (e.g., viable epidermis, dermis, fat, or appendages). The rate and extent of binding have only been documented for a few compounds, but the methodology appears to be adequate. Toxic agents presumably bind to several tissue compartments. Chemical defensive agents might saturate binding sites to decrease the toxicity of the attacking agent.

Anatomic Pathways

Penetration occurs throughout the stratum corneum. Empirically, it is known that hairy areas (terminal or vellus hairs) are more permeable than glabrous sites (e.g., the retroauricular area, face, scalp, and axilla are more permeable than the forearm). Understanding the mechanisms controlling these differences might provide insights for chemical defense.

Cutaneous Metabolism

The skin is an extremely active metabolic organ that contains numerous chemical-metabolizing enzymes. Metabolism of a chemical in skin may alter the pharmacological and/or toxicological effect on the system. When studying the availability of topically administered drugs or environmental contaminants, one must consider the metabolizing ability of the skin, which may affect the bioavailability of the drug during the first passage through the skin. For example, hydrocortisone can be metabolized to cortisone and dihydrodiols can be metabolized to expoxide diols, which are more potent carcinogens than the original chemicals.

Evaluation of Barrier Creams

Recently, DPD models and noninvasive bioengineering techniques have been adapted to quantify the efficacy of protective or decontaminating barrier creams. These tests provide accurate, reproducible, and objective observations that can reveal subtle differences before visual clinical signs (e.g., blisters) appear (Berardesca et al., 1995a, 1995b; Elsner et al., 1994; Frosch et al., 1993a; Wilhelm et al., 1997). These tests are considered to be more humane than traditional tests because, by the time a blister develops after vesicant exposure, critical biological events have occurred. Data on the efficacy of barrier creams from recent experiments are summarized in Table 6-1. The *in vivo* and *in vitro* methods used to evaluate barrier creams are provided in Appendix C.

TEST EQUIPMENT

Because the United States has moved to a joint service environment and adheres to the CWC and the BWC, testing has become a complicated issue in two respects. First, simulant agents that mimic the chemical and physical properties of real agents must be used. Second, responsibilities must be distributed across services. For example, the Marine Corps is responsible for testing JSLIST but does not "own" the expertise for performing these tests; the toxicological expertise resides in the Army at SBCCOM Soldier Systems Center. The U.S. Army Chemical School (now relocated to Ft. Leonard Wood) has the capability to conduct exercises using real chemical agents, but such experiments are limited to training exercises. Army facilities cannot be used for testing components of PPE or ensembles, per se (DoD, 1999).

PPE components and ensembles have been tested by contract personnel at Dugway Proving Ground in Utah using simulants. The Dugway facilities have excellent capabilities (1) for testing with CB simulants, such as methyl salycilate (MES), which is environmentally benign and relatively nontoxic; (2) for large-scale field testing of the integrity, degree of protection, and decontamination of PPE; and (3) for modeling exercises using various exposure scenarios. Unfortunately, although the capability for performing quantitative tests is available, no mechanism has been established for coordinating the toxicological, human factors, and exposure assessments of the studies.

The lack of coordination becomes apparent in a review of the studies

TABLE 6-1 Efficacy of Barrier Creams

Models		
In Vitro	*In Vivo* Animals or Human	Irritants or Allergens
	Guinea pigs	n-Hexane, trichloroethylene, and toluene
	Guinea pigs	cutting oil
	Humans with a history of allergic reactions to test allergens	epoxy resin, glyceryl monothioglycolate, frullania, and tansy
	Humans who had positive patch tests to toxicodendron extract	toxicodendron extract
	Guinea pigs and humans	sodium lauryl sulfate, sodium hydroxide, toluene, and lactic acid
Human skin		dyes (eosin, methylviolet, oil red O)
	Machinists	Castrol oil
	Humans with a history of allergic reaction to poison ivy/oak	urushiol
	Nickel-sensitive patients	nickel disc
	Humans	dyes (methylene blue and oil red O)

Barrier Cream	Efficacy	References
3 water-miscible creams	Had limited protective effects.	Mahmoud and Lachapelle, 1985
2 barrier creams	Exacerbated the irritation.	Goh, 1991a, 1991b
1 barrier cream	Minimized the development of allergic contact dermatitis.	McClain and Storrs, 1992
various barrier preparations	Most provided good protective effects.	Grevelink et al., 1992
several barrier creams	Some suppressed irritation, some failed, and some caused severe irritation.	Frosch et al., 1993b, 1993c, 1993d; Frosch and Kurte, 1994
16 barrier creams	Various protection effects.	Treffel et al., 1994
1 barrier cream and 1 afterwork emollient	Had no significant effect against dermatitis from cutting fluid.	Goh and Gan, 1994
quaternium-18 bentonite (Q18B) lotion	Significantly reduced reactions.	Marks et al., 1995
ethylenediamine-tetra-acetate (EDTA) gels	Significantly reduced the amount of nickel in the epidermis *in vitro*, and significantly reduced positive reactions *in vivo*.	Fullerton and Menne, 1995
3 barrier creams	Two creams were effective, one increased the cumulative amount of dye.	Zhai and Maibach, 1996

TABLE 6-1 Efficacy of Barrier Creams (continued)

Models		
In Vitro	In Vivo Animals or Human	Irritants or Allergens
	Humans	water
	Humans	10% sodium lauryl sulfate, 1% NaOH, 30% lactic acid, and undiluted toluene
	Humans	toluene
	Humans	toluene and NaOH
	Guinea pigs	sulphur mustard
	Humans	self-application of barrier cream
Human skin		[^{35}S]-SLS
	Humans	sodium lauryl sulfate, ammonium hydroxide (NH$_4$OH), urea, Rhus

Barrier Cream	Efficacy	References
2 barrier creams and a moisturizer	Various protection effects.	Olivarius et al., 1996
4 barrier creams and white petrolatum	Had different protective effects but all products were very effective against SLS.	Schlüter-Wigger and Elsner, 1996
several barrier creams	All markedly reduced the effect of repetitive toluene contact.	Grunewald et al., 1996
several barrier creams	None prevented the skin erythema induced by toluene. One barrier cream, as well as petrolatum and a fatty cream, protected the skin significantly against NaOH.	Treffel and Gabard, 1996
povidone iodine (PI) ointment	Showed powerful protective effect.	Wormser et al., 1997
oil-in-water emulsion	Self-application was incomplete.	Wigger-Alberti et al., 1997
3 quaternium-18, bentonite (Q18B), gels	Protection effects were 88%, 81%, and 65%, respectively.	Zhai et al., 1999
several protectants	Most suppressed the SLS irritation and Rhus allergic reaction, but did not suppress NH_4OH and urea irritation.	Zhai et al., 1998

referred to as the Man-in-Simulant Test (MIST) Program. Despite its shortcomings (described below), MIST is an extremely valuable program that has the potential to test complete and partial PPE ensembles under controlled field conditions. A series of tests in which individuals were exposed to MES at a steady-state concentration of 100 mg/m^3 for a period of two hours provided a useful "reality check" (NRC, 1997b). As is often necessary in field-testing situations, however, compromises had to be made. In the MIST ensemble testing, the PPE components were worn and compared with standard issue uniforms. As the test progressed, some of the PPE were damaged. Of these, some were repaired and reworn, while others were worn without repair. Although this is probably what would happen in real-world use, the initial protocol was degraded, thus compromising the use of the data to predict what would happen if PPE were used in a contaminated environment during an actual field deployment.

Another problem with the MIST study was that the comparability of MES to H or V agents was not taken fully into account. Thus, the MIST review committee judged that the MIST data might be used qualitatively to rank some types of PPE, but that the data could not be used to make quantitative assessments because the information obtained using the passive dosimeters (i.e., samplers) could not be correlated to the amount of H or V agents that contacted the skin.

Based on the assumption that MES was a reasonable surrogate for H agents, the test data showed the following results:

- Under the most favorable conditions (PPE in excellent condition), the complete ensemble provided protection against a challenge of $\leq 3,000$ mg-min/m^3.
- Damage to the ensemble during use degraded performance to a challenge capability of ≤ 500 mg-min/m^3.
- Ensembles that were damaged, repaired, or reworn provided protection against a challenge of ≤ 500 mg-min/m^3.
- The areas of greatest vulnerability in an intact PPE are seals and closures.
- The passive dosimeters used to test other components of the protective equipment did not function reliably in the mask.

Because of problems in the experimental design, the data on protection afforded by PPE ensembles could only be used in a qualitative way. Nevertheless, they can still be very useful. For example, the data showed that, within the limits of statistical error, the BDO did not afford significantly greater protection than chemical protective undergarments. This apparent anomaly is attributable to the large differences among ensemble components.

The MIST study might be considered a pilot study for more definitive future studies. The data from the MIST study could be used to design a stronger statistical study based on the basic science aspects of using simulants, such as MES, to determine whether or not PPE ensembles provide adequate protection against challenges with CB agents (or suitable simulants). To facilitate the selection of suppliers of materials, closures, and other parts of the PPE ensemble, the tests should be designed to compare the performance of various ensembles (or components). At a minimum, better methods for validating the use of simulants will be necessary so that results can be used quantitatively. This may require better coordination among groups at SBCCOM and Dugway Proving Ground.

Current mask filters are extremely efficient and afford adequate protection under expected challenge conditions. The point of failure in respiratory protection is the mask seal, not the filter cartridge. The MIST Program did not test masks because the passive monitors used to detect MES and the mask systems were incompatible. This problem has not yet been resolved.

PREDICTIVE MODELS AND SIMULATIONS

Modeling and simulation are often used in place of prototyping to predict the operational characteristics of protective systems. Current models, however, may not be robust or reliable enough to use for making crucial decisions. A major problem is the lack of basic science information, such as the persistence of agents in various environments and under various conditions, rates of deposition, uptake and metabolism in living human skin, and rates of penetration under realistic conditions.

EXERCISES AND SYSTEMS EVALUATIONS

Various types of exercises are used to evaluate the ability of deployed and deploying forces to operate in a CB environment. Computer exercises and war games can be used to predict the likely behavior and effects of operating in a CB environment. The accuracy of the predictions depends on the quality of the data used in the computer model parameter estimates. Computerized war games and scenarios, such as CB2010 (a simulation of the effects of a "low-tech" CB attack on a U.S. force during deployment from a base in CONUS in the year 2010) predicted that a CB attack would significantly impact force projection capabilities, especially the speed of deployment and the effectiveness of forces. A subsequent, more realistic war game with a similar scenario was "played" during a deployment exercise at Pope Air Force Base and Fort Bragg. The actual effects of spraying a simulated thickened mustard on mission-critical equipment and service areas from a crop-duster-type aircraft demonstrated that the computer simulation might have been optimistic. The impacts were more protracted and additional problems were identified.

FINDINGS AND RECOMMENDATIONS

Finding. Testing of dermatological threat agents has not been consistent. The available data are not sufficiently precise to make an accurate evaluation of potential percutaneous threats from agents other than blister agents or irritants.

Recommendation. Tests of dermatological threat agents should be conducted to establish the level of protection necessary to provide adequate margins of safety and to establish quantitative criteria for evaluating the performance of protective equipment, such as gloves, undergarments, and overgarments.

Finding. Mask testing under the MIST program was unreliable because the passive dosimeters did not function satisfactorily.

Recommendation. Active samplers or improved passive samplers for mask testing using simulants should be developed and made available for tests of the joint service lightweight integrated suit technology (JSLIST) ensemble.

7

Assessment of Military Capabilities to Provide Emergency Response

In a sense, the subject of military emergency response capabilities in civil situations is beyond the scope of this study, which is focused on deployed forces. However, because the agencies responsible for the protection of our forces also have certain responsibilities during domestic CB terrorist incidents, this subject is treated briefly.

Because of recent concerns about possible CB terrorist incidents in the United States, various initiatives have been implemented and numerous studies undertaken to assess emergency response capabilities (e.g., GAO, 1999; IOM, 1999b). Many of these initiatives define the role of the U.S. military in coordination with other federal (e.g., the Federal Bureau of Investigation, the Federal Emergency Management Agency, the U.S. Department of Energy), state, and local agencies.

For example, the Domestic Preparedness Initiative, established in the FY 1997 Defense Authorization Bill (Public Law 104-201), commonly referred to as the Nunn-Lugar-Domenici legislation, provides funding for DoD to enhance the capabilities of federal, state, and local emergency responders in incidents involving NBC terrorism. In response, SBCCOM has set up a hot line to provide emergency responders and emergency planners with immediate access to information during a CB terrorist incident. SBCCOM also provides training to improve existing metropolitan response capabilities to CB incidents.

The Army has formed specialty response teams to complement the military medical response in the event of a local, national, or international CB attack. The two teams, which are required to be capable of deploying within 18 to 24 hours of notification, are the Special Medical Augmentation

Response Team-Preventative Medicine (SMART-PM) and the Special Medical Augmentation Response Team-Chemical/Biological (SMART-CB). The mission of the SMART-PM team is to provide initial assessments of disease and environmental health threats either prior to or in the initial stages of a contingency operation or during the early or continuing stages of a disaster.

The SMART-CB includes the National Medical Chemical-Biological Advisory Team (MCBAT) and the Regional Medical Command CB Specialty Response Teams (CB-SRTs). SMART CB components, which are elements of the DoD Chemical Biological Rapid Response Team, are required to be ready to deploy worldwide within four hours of receiving their orders. The responsibilities of the National MCBAT and the regional CB-SRT include: (1) providing medical advice to commanders or local authorities (a) on protecting first responders and other health care personnel, (b) on casualty decontamination procedures, and (c) on first aid and initial medical treatment; and (2) aiding in handling casualties.

USAMRICD has developed a Chemical Casualty Site Team with the capability of rapid deployment in support of DoD, the Foreign Emergency Response Team, or the Domestic Emergency Response Team. The personnel available for deployment can provide information on the medical effects of specific chemical warfare agents, identify chemical agents or their metabolites in biological samples, determine blood cholinesterase levels, provide technical and biomedical means to protect personnel responding to chemical incidents or to decontaminate personnel and casualties, and assist with mission planning. Military units can also provide training, advice, and assistance in bomb disposal and decontamination operations.

A 350-member Marine Corps unit, the Chemical Biological Incident Response Force (CBIRF), assists with evacuation, decontamination, and medical stabilization of victims. CBIRF is required to be able to have an advance party airborne within four hours of notification; however, given its limitations, this unit is likely to play a major role only when deployed to a site in advance (e.g., the 1996 Olympics in Atlanta) (IOM, 1999b).

Recently, the Army published a regulation stating that U.S. Army medical treatment facilities and clinics will provide assistance to civilian first responders in the event of a CB terrorist act and emergency room and in-patient treatment for both DoD beneficiaries and civilian casualties (U.S. Army, 1998). Requirements of the Surgeon General include: coordinating emergency medical CB response capabilities worldwide with other DoD, joint service, federal, state, local, and host nation agencies; maintaining medical CB response teams to address emerging infectious diseases and chemical accidents/incidents worldwide; and establishing policy and guidelines for managing and treating conventional and CB casualties.

The National Guard has established rapid assessment and initial detection (RAID) teams in 10 areas around the country (designated by the Federal Emergency Management Agency) to respond to terrorist attacks in the United States that involve CB agents. These teams are designated to be the first military responders sent to help civilian authorities detect and assess CB agents. They are also prepared to train local authorities in CB weapons detection, defense, and decontamination; assist in casualty treatment and evacuation; quarantine affected areas and people; and assist in restoration of infrastructure and services.

Many recommendations have recently been made to improve U.S. readiness to respond (e.g., GAO, 1999; IOM, 1999b), and initial efforts have been made to implement some of them. For example, to protect civilian emergency responders in the event of a CB warfare incident, the National Institute for Occupational Safety and Health (NIOSH), the SBCCOM, and the Occupational Safety and Health Administration are working together to provide respiratory protection for emergency responders. Currently, respiratory protection that is certified by NIOSH for use against CB agents is not available.

Much less attention, however, has been given to responding to CB attacks against U.S. facilities on foreign soil. Although many safeguards have been put in place since the attacks on the U.S. embassies in Kenya and Tanzania in October 1998, others have been identified and have been, or are in the process of being, added. In general, the U.S. Department of State and the Federal Bureau of Investigation are primarily responsible for dealing with these types of incidents; however, the host nation often provides medical treatment and works with the United States in response to the attack. Documentation obtained during the course of this study did not include the role of the military in these types of attacks.

Based on a presentation about the proposed NATO Long-Term Scientific Study on Chemical and Biological Defense (Medema, 1999), there are significant deficiencies in doctrine and guidance for emergency responses in allied countries. No provisions are being made to ensure that host nation forces are equipped with CB protective equipment compatible with the equipment used by U.S. forces. Nor are there provisions for training foreign nationals engaged in mission-critical activities on U.S. bases in host nations that might be targets for CB attack.

FINDINGS AND RECOMMENDATIONS

Finding. Because numerous agencies will respond to a domestic CB incident, close cooperation will be necessary for the response to be efficient and effective. Unless civilians (e.g., first responders, employees of relevant state and local agencies, etc.) who respond to domestic CB incidents are equipped with protective and decontamination equipment that is compatible with equipment used by the military, coordination will be difficult if not impossible.

Recommendation. The Department of Defense, in collaboration with civilian agencies, should provide compatible equipment and training to civilians (e.g., first responders, employees of relevant state and local agencies, etc.) who respond to domestic chemical and/or biological incidents to ensure that their activities can be coordinated with the activities of military units. Doctrine and guidance should be developed on an interagency basis.

Finding. Doctrine and training are not well developed for mission-critical civilians working at military installations that might become targets of chemical and/or biological attacks.

Recommendation. Coordinated doctrine, training, and guidance on individual protective equipment, collective protective equipment, and decontamination for civilians working at military installations should be established on a joint service, interagency and coalition basis.

8

Summary and General Recommendations

Since the demise of the Soviet Union and the breakdown of the Warsaw Pact, a number of events have influenced the way the United States plans to protect against CB attacks:

- Stronger ties have been formed between NATO and Eastern European nations.
- The Gulf War was successfully prosecuted, but there are lingering questions about whether illnesses reported by returning personnel resulted from undetected exposure to CB agents.
- Terrorists have used and threatened to use CB agents.
- The United States has agreed to adhere to the precepts of the CWC and the BWC.
- CB weapon technology has been proliferating.
- New techniques in molecular biosciences have increased the potential threat of biological weapons.
- In the future, it is probable that a larger number of biological and chemical agents will be available, which will broaden the threat.
- For the foreseeable future, the acceptance rate of U.S. casualties from CB exposures is likely to remain very low.

The health of military personnel who served in the Gulf War, as well as of personnel who will participate in future deployments, is a matter of great concern to veterans, the public, Congress, and DoD. Based on the lessons learned from the Gulf War and subsequent deployments, as well as other evidence that has accrued, potential adverse health effects to U.S.

forces from exposure to CB agents can be minimized and protection levels increased.

This report focuses on (1) an assessment and evaluation of approaches and technologies that are, or might be, used by DoD in the development and evaluation of clothing and equipment for physical protection and decontamination; and (2) an assessment of current policies, doctrine, and training as they relate to protection against exposure and decontamination after exposure to CB agents.

THREAT

Threat projections are developed and validated by the intelligence community based on data from military and civilian intelligence agencies. These data are then used by the military to focus R&D and to develop policy and doctrine (and by extension tactics and training) and to define equipment parameters (requirements and specifications).

During the Cold War, Soviet Forces were believed to possess a broad range of CB weapons and to have the capability of deploying and supporting those weapons on the battlefield. The Soviet Union was also believed to be pursuing an extensive CB R&D program. The threat projections provided by the intelligence community included lists of delivery systems, agents, the weaponization of agents, and R&D programs that could lead to the weaponization of novel agents.

The Soviet Union was credited with having a stockpile of CB weapons and the tactical and logistical capabilities to saturate a battle space with agents. The knowledge that the Soviet Union had created a large CB decontamination force and included CB challenges in its training supported the belief that the Soviets could mount and sustain a battlefield-scale CB attack.

In addition, the knowledge that the Soviet Union was committing major resources to R&D and that design bureaus were focused on developing CB weaponry heightened the expectation that U.S. forces might encounter novel CB agents on the battlefield. Although information on the specific nature of these agents was sparse, it was widely believed that the protective clothing and masks available and distributed to U.S. troops would not provide adequate protection against the potentially vast array of these hitherto unknown agents.

Based on the belief that the Soviets had significant CB weapons and research capabilities, the requirements for protective equipment were more stringent than might have been necessary, even for use on a battlefield awash in known agents. Even though the Soviet Union has now been dismantled, current U.S. R&D is based on the same rigorous design criteria for protective equipment, partly because of uncertainties about threats from potential adversaries, but also because of the prevailing view that casualties from exposures to CB agents are simply not acceptable.

POLICY, DOCTRINE, AND TRAINING

In keeping with the ideas described above, current U.S. tactics and training are based on a doctrine of contamination avoidance. The amount and intensity of training, however, have been left to the discretion of individual commanders, who are also responsible for assessing the effectiveness of training.

The requirements for training and protective equipment are based on the challenge expected on the battlefield. The CB challenge can be defined as the numerical limits on the CB environment where deployed personnel must operate. Ballistic threat levels might be defined in terms of speed, momentum, and the physical properties of a projectile. CB threat levels are defined in terms of the concentration of agent in which operations must take place over a period of time.

For chemical agents in liquid form, the challenge is most often described in terms of liquid mass/area measured over time. Vaporous agent challenges are defined as concentration measured over time. In general, the liquid chemical agent challenge has been set at $10 g/m^2$ for 24 hours for all agents, and the vaporous chemical agent challenge has been between 5,000 mg-min/m^3 and 10,000 mg-min/m^3.

Definitions of biological agent challenges are generally based on LD_{50}s and minimum infective doses for individual agents. Therefore, the challenges of various agents vary greatly. However, it is generally assumed in the CB community that equipment that provides 24 hour, 10 g/m^2 protection against liquid chemical agent will also provide protection against biological agents. Although this may be true for respiratory protection, it may not be true for biological aerosols that pose a percutaneous threat. Tests of protective ensembles against aerosol threats have not been extensive enough to establish protection factors.

CHEMICAL/BIOLOGICAL PROTECTIVE EQUIPMENT

Once doctrine, tactics, and training have been established, equipment must be developed to support CB defense. The R&D process used for CB protective equipment has changed significantly over time.

Threat-Based Requirements and the Development of Equipment

Based on widespread perceptions of Soviet CB stockpiles, troop training, and weapons capabilities, the design requirements for protective equipment were to withstand a liquid agent challenge of 10 g/m² for 24 hours. Similarly high (service-specific and agent-specific) challenges for vaporous chemical agents were set. In other words, it was anticipated that a battle space could be virtually awash in chemical agents. These design requirements have not been substantially revised since the dissolution of the Soviet Union.

Recent analyses of liquid agent deposition using relatively sophisticated computer models have determined that under some conditions 10 g/m² levels are possible in localized areas of a battlefield (although the average concentration may be considerably lower). However, these same models predict that the areas of high concentration would coincide with areas where shrapnel and projected shell materials would be more likely to injure or kill personnel than CB agents. Based on computer modeling, some troops may be required to enter highly contaminated areas to recover injured personnel and move them to medical facilities or to relocate mission-critical equipment from a contaminated area to a decontamination zone. In general, however, the number of individuals in areas with contamination near the 10 g/m² level will be small, and the duration of their exposure will be short.

Challenge levels not only determine requirements for protection, they also influence tactics and training. Apparently, the tactics, training, and requirements for CB defense have not changed significantly since the demise of the Soviet Union, although the threat to U.S. forces has changed in the following ways:

- No potentially hostile proliferant country has an R&D structure as capable of producing novel CB weapons as the Soviet Union. Therefore, a surprise attack with novel chemical agents is much less likely than it was. In fact, attacks with unanticipated biological agents are more likely than attacks with unanticipated chemical agents.
- The intelligence community is generally capable of assessing the character of threats posed by current hostile proliferant nations.
- No hostile proliferant nation has the resources or capability to mount a substantial research program or to pose a significant battlefield challenge to U.S. troops.
- CB challenges to deployed forces will probably occur in operations other than war.
- CB challenges to deployed forces could occur as low-level exposures.

The current protection level for CB threats (100 percent) is higher than the protection level for ballistic threats. Therefore, the selection of protection factors has been extremely conservative, and the design criteria for protective equipment are probably more restrictive than necessary. As a result, the development of equipment has been slow and costly.

The detrimental effects of wearing protective equipment on troop performance may also have been unnecessarily increased because of requirements imposed to meet the stringent challenge levels. Results of tests on clothing and equipment for effects on individual and unit effectiveness, as well as requirements for CB protection, should be considered in a coordinated way so that design criteria are optimized for providing protection and minimizing performance degradations. Protective equipment with less detrimental effects on individual and unit effectiveness could be developed if equipment requirements were based on more realistic challenges. In general, the expectation that individual and collective protective equipment can provide 100 percent protection against CB challenges is unrealistic.

Recommendation. Threat projections and risk perceptions should be reevaluated in terms of realistic, up-to-date battlefield risks. The requirements for protective equipment should then be adjusted to respond to those threats and challenges.

Many questions remain unanswered about how to characterize low-level contamination. This problem resurfaced with questions about the health problems of Gulf War veterans, which many believe are the results of exposures to CB agents or other potentially harmful substances (e.g., environmental and occupational contaminants and toxic industrial chemicals) during their deployment. Knowledge of the effects of extended exposures to low levels of CB agents is incomplete, but recent studies suggest that there may be some long-term consequences of low-level exposures. Requirements for protection against percutaneous threats are based on these definitions, however, as are the goals of the R&D program.

Recommendation. Research on the toxicology of low-level, long-term exposures to chemical and biological agents and other potentially harmful substances (e.g., environmental and occupational contaminants and toxic industrial chemicals) should be continued and expanded.

Physical Protection

Specific vulnerabilities, such as the seals of protective masks against the face and suit overlap and closure points, should be given high priority. In this report, various materials for protective clothing, mask seals, mask filters, and protective gloves and boots materials were reviewed, and future directions for materials research were suggested. The development of protective gear in response to unreasonably high projected challenges has led to the fielding of protective gear that is unduly cumbersome and interferes with performance. Training in mask fit testing and the proper use of MOPP gear are not uniform across or within the services.

Masks, garments, gloves, and boots were designed as independent items and then "retrofitted" to create an ensemble. They were also developed without adequate attention to various human factors, issues such as the integration of the protective gear with weapon systems.

Recommendation. A total systems analysis, including human factors engineering evaluations, should be part of the development process of the personal protective equipment system to ensure that the protective equipment can be used with weapon systems and other military equipment. These evaluations should include the following aspects:

- the performance of individuals and units on tasks in different various realistic scenarios
- the interface of the mask with garments and potential leakage during an "advance" from Mask-Only status to MOPP 4 status

Recommendation. Additional research should be done on mask seals and mask fit. The research program should focus on seals, fit, and sealants (adhesives). In addition, training for properly fitting masks should be provided for all deployed forces equipped with mission-oriented protective posture (MOPP) equipment.

Decontamination

Most current decontamination systems are labor and resource intensive, require excessive amounts of water, are corrosive and/or toxic, and are not considered environmentally safe. Current R&D is aimed at developing decontamination systems that would overcome these limitations and effectively decontaminate a broad spectrum of CB agents from all surfaces and materials. DoD has developed doctrine and training protocols for the use of decontaminants, but in order to relate doctrine to risk, guidelines must first be established for what constitutes acceptable risk. Although some of the elements necessary for developing appropriate guidance exist, there are still deficiencies. (For example, detection capabilities are not designed for the decontamination environment, and few benchmarks have been established for determining the effectiveness of decontamination.)

Recommendation. Joint service, interagency, and multinational standards should be established for decontamination levels. These standards should be based on the best science available and may require the development of new models for setting standards, especially for highly toxic or pathogenic agents.

Testing

Testing equipment and determining the physiological effects of individual agents are important factors in the development of requirements for equipment. Simulants are commonly used to test protective and decontamination equipment. However, the degree to which the behavior of simulants mimics the behavior of real agents has not been well established. Therefore, based on simulant testing, it is difficult to determine whether or not a specific piece of equipment has met its performance requirements.

In general, knowledge of the physiological effects of CB agents is based on animal studies, anecdotal evidence, and random accidents. Estimated percutaneous threats from chemical agents are based mostly on animal studies; while estimated percutaneous threats from biological agents are based mostly on anecdotal evidence. Because the requirements for protection against percutaneous threats are based on data that has limited applicability, the goals, requirements, and results of the R&D programs are necessarily based on uncertainties.

Recommendation. The use of simulants, data from animal models, and data on human exposure should be reevaluated as part of the development of a coherent research program to determine the physiological effects of both high-level and low-level long-term exposures to chemical and biological agents. The data should then be used to determine risks and challenges.

Use of modeling and simulation may be a partial solution to the paucity of data. However, in the case of CB protective equipment, little evidence indicates that modeling and simulation are effective.

Even if the protective equipment were 100 percent effective, inconsistent and inadequate training virtually guarantees that it will not be properly used. The methods for determining the effectiveness of training, especially in the joint service environment, have not been well defined. Until objective criteria are developed, the quality of current and planned training cannot be assessed.

Recommendation. Required levels of training (with the appropriate level of funding for training devices and simulants) should be established and monitored for effective unit performance throughout the services. Objective criteria should be established for determining whether current service-specific training requirements are being met.

Program Objective Memorandum for Funding Research

The primary approach to CB defense, according to current doctrine, is contamination avoidance, which depends primarily on the detection of contamination. Therefore, detection technologies should have the highest priority in terms of investment and, by inference, in terms of R&D. R&D should focus first on detection, then on protection, and then on decontamination.

Although parsing out the individual investment strategies supporting the POM figures is difficult, the basic strategy should reflect the following philosophy:

- Contamination avoidance requires knowing where agent has been deposited, how much agent is present, and how long the agent has been (and will be) present.
- Challenge levels should be adjusted in accordance with current understanding of the potential threat, and design criteria for protective equipment should be revised accordingly.
- The mask is the single most important component of the individual's protective ensemble because it protects the most vulnerable systems (respiratory system, eyes, and digestive system).
- Protective clothing (including boots and gloves) are secondary to the mask.
- Collective protective equipment has been developed, but few units have been fielded.
- Given realistic battle space threats and the emphasis on contamination avoidance, the need for decontamination of mobile forces should be reduced, but the need for decontamination doctrine, training, and equipment for fixed sites may be increased.

Recommendation. Funding priorities in the Program Objective Memorandum should reflect the following priorities:

1. point and remote detection of chemical and biological agents
2. rigorous development and validation of simulants for testing protective equipment

3. improvements in mask seals and fit
4. improvements in protective clothing
5. improvements in gloves and boots
6. decontamination technologies

SUMMARY

Although substantial improvements have been made in the protection of deployed forces from CB agents, progress has been hampered by overly conservative design criteria for equipment based on challenges that may not be credible today. In addition, substantial changes have been made in the way military missions will be prosecuted (e.g., force projection, joint service requirements, expanded use of reserve troops, adherence to the CWC and BWC), but the development of doctrine and guidelines has not kept pace. However, recent efforts by the United States, as well as NATO, are addressing these problems.

Many problems remain to be solved in the development of systematic protocols for testing protective equipment, both in terms of experimental design and in the selection of appropriate surrogates for agents. In addition, a total systems analysis (including human factors engineering), not just component testing, should be conducted as new component design criteria are imposed to minimize cognitive and physical performance degradations.

The best equipment can fail, however, if users are not properly trained. Appropriate training on methods of donning and removing protective gear, as well as training for commanders in decision making when a CB threat is encountered, will increase the likelihood that U.S. forces will use the equipment they have correctly, and thus, increase the probability of successfully completing their mission, even under CB conditions.

References

Albizo, J.M., J.W. Hovanec, and J.R. Ward. 1988. Decontamination of Organophosphorous Esters by Hydrolysis Catalyzed by Transition-Metal Ions. CRDEC-TR-88061. Aberdeen Proving Ground, Md.: Chemical Research Development and Engineering.

Ali, J., L. Rodrigues, and M. Moodie. 1997. U.S. Chemical-Biological Defense Guidebook. Alexandria, Va.: Jane's Information Group.

ARO (Army Research Office). 1997. MURI/ARO Functionally Tailored Textile Fabrics. Interim Progress Report. DAAH04-96-1-0018. Research Triangle Park, N.C.: Army Research Office.

ASTM (American Society for Testing and Materials). 1993. Designation ES 22-92. Emergency standard test method for resistance to protective clothing materials to penetration by blood-borne pathogens using viral penetration as a test system. Annual Book of ASTM Standards 11.03: 807.

Bannard, R.A.B., A.A. Casselman, J.G. Purdon, and J.W. Bovenkamp. 1991. U.S. Patent no. 5,077,316. 1991 December 31.

Barrett, G. 1998. PM-ESS (Enhanced Soldier Systems) Managed Programs. Presentation by G. Barrett, Program Manager, Enhanced Soldier Systems, to principal investigators and members of the Advisory Panel on Strategies to Protect the Health of Deployed U.S. Forces, Task 2.3: Physical Protection and Decontamination. Soldier and Biological Chemical Command, Natick, Massachusetts, November 16, 1999.

Bartram, P.W., V.D. Henderson, J.W. Hovanec, M.D. Brickhouse, and G.W. Wagner. 1998. Reactions of GD and VX with Ozone. Final Report TR-550. Abingdon, Md.: EAI Corporation.

Battelle Memorial Institute and Charles Williams, Inc. 1999. Chemical and Biological Wide Area Decontamination Literature Search and Market Survey. Report to the Joint Service Materiel Group. Bel Air, Md.: Battelle Memorial Institute.

Beaudry, W.T., L.L. Szafraniec, and D.R. Leslie. 1990. Sorption and Reaction of Organophosphorus Compounds by a Mixed Sorbtive/Reactive Resin. Pp. 91–98 in Proceedings of the 1990 Edgewood Research, Development, and Engineering Center Scientific Conference on Chemical Defense Research. Aberdeen Proving Ground, Md.: Edgewood Research, Development, and Engineering Center.

REFERENCES

Bell, W.L., S.D. Dietz, S.C. Gebhard, G.R. Mason, T.J. Selegue, and P.M. Nolan. 1998. Novel Carbonaceous Sorbants. Pp. 461–467 in Proceedings of the 1997 Edgewood Research, Development, and Engineering Center Scientific Conference on Chemical Defense Research. November 18–21, 1997, Aberdeen Proving Ground, Md. Edgewood Research, Development, and Engineering Center.

Berardesca, E., P. Elsner, K.P. Wilhelm, and H.I. Maibach. 1995a. Bioengineering of the Skin: Methods and Instrumentation. Boca Raton, Fla.: CRC Press.

Berardesca, E., P. Elsner, and H.I. Maibach. 1995b. Bioengineering of the Skin: Cutaneous Blood Flow and Erythema. Boca Raton, Fla.: CRC Press.

Blankenbiller, A. 1998. Overview of the JSMG. Presentation by A. Blankenbiller, Program Manager, Joint Research and Development, to principal investigators on Strategies to Protect the Health of Deployed U.S. Forces, Task 2.3: Physical Protection and Decontamination, National Research Council, Washington, D.C., April 28, 1998.

Bloomfield, S.F., and M. Arther. 1992. Interaction of *Bacillus subtilis* spores with sodium hypochlorite, sodium dichloroisocyanorate and chloramine-T. Journal of Applied Bacteriology 72: 166.

Bolton, J.R., and R.D.S. Stevens. 1995. The Potential for UV-Based Advanced Oxidation Processes for the Destruction of Chemical Warfare Agents. Pp. 347–358 in Proceedings of the Workshop on Advances in Alternative Demilitarization Technologies. Washington, D.C.: U.S. Army.

Booz-Allen and Hamilton. 1997. Assessment of the Impact of Chemical and Biological Weapons on Joint Operations in 2010 (The CB 2010 Study). McLean, Va.: Booz-Allen and Hamilton.

Boyle, R.E. 1998a. Biological Warfare: A Historical Perspective. LG-1597. Albuquerque, N.M.: Sandia National Laboratories.

Boyle, R.E. 1998b. U.S. Chemical Warfare: A Historical Perspective. LG-1597. Albuquerque, N.M.: Sandia National Laboratories.

Brandler, P. 1998. State-of-the-Art of Functional Textiles for Soldiers' Related Systems, Functionally Tailored Textiles and Fabrics. Presented at the Second Annual Review Meeting. Army Research Laboratories, Aberdeen, Md., March 5–6, 1998.

Braue, E.H., Jr. 1998. Development of a Reactive Topical Skin Protectant. Presentation by E.H. Braue, Jr., to the Decontamination Commodity Area Program Review Meeting, Joint Service Materiel Group, Edgewood, Maryland, October 7–8, 1998.

Buettner, L.C., L.E. Campbell, S.S. Hsu, J.T. James, C.J. Karwacki, S.A. Katz, R.W. Morrison, and W.T. Muse. 1988. An Experimental Assessment of Protective Filters Challenged by Toxic Gases Potentially Present in the Bradley Fighting Vehicle. CRDEC-TR-88096. Aberdeen Proving Ground, Md.: U.S. Army.

Bunton, C.A., G. Cerichelli, Y. Ihara, and L. Sepulveda. 1979. Micellar catalysis and reactant incorporation in dephosphorylation and nucleophilic substitution. Journal of the American Chemical Society 101: 2429–2435.

Bunton, C.A., F.D. Buzzaccarini, and F.H. Hamed. 1983. Nucleophilic aromatic-substitution in microemulsions of hydroxyethyl surfactants. Journal of Organic Chemistry 48(15): 2461–2465.

Bunton, C.A., and C. Quan. 1985. Hydrolysis of 2,4-dinitrophenyl phosphate in hydrophobic ammonium-salts. Journal of Organic Chemistry 50: 3230–3232.

Bunton, C.A., M.M. Mhala, and J.R. Moffatt. 1990. Dephosphorylation by peroxyanions in micelles and microemulsions. Journal of Physical Organic Chemistry 3: 390–396.

Bunton, C.A., and H.J. Foroudian. 1993. A quantitative treatment of micellar effects upon dephosphorylation by hydroperoxide anion. Langmuir 9: 2832–2835.

Cag, P., H. Dobbs, R. Herz, B. Liu, and D. Woodrum. 1995. Integration of Catalytic Oxidation/Environmental Control Unit (CATOX/ECU) Air Purification System into Combat Vehicle. ERDEC-CR-175. Aberdeen Proving Ground, Md.: U.S. Army.

Cain, E. 1999. Biological Defense Program Review. Presentation by E. Cain, Joint Program Manager for Biological Defense, Joint Program Office (Biological Defense) to the Department of Defense Nuclear, Biological, and Chemical Symposium and Exhibition. Aberdeen Proving Ground, Maryland, June 22, 1999.

Calomiris, J.J., T. Cheng, S.P. Harvey, and J.J. DeFrank. 1994. Enzymatic Catalysis of Organophosphorus Toxicants. Pp. 919–925 in Proceedings of the 1993 Edgewood Research, Development, and Engineering Center Scientific Conference on Chemical Defense Research, November 16–19, 1993. Aberdeen Proving Ground, Md.: Edgewood Research, Development, and Engineering Center.

Carr, J.L., B.M. Corona, S.E. Jackson, and V.L. Bachovchin. 1980a. The effects of chemical biological clothing and equipment on U.S. Army soldiers' performance: a critical review of the literature (a preliminary survey). Technical Memorandum 12-80. Aberdeen Proving Ground, Md.: U.S. Army Human Engineering Laboratory.

Carr, J.L., R.L. Kershner, B.M. Corona, and S.E. Jackson. 1980b. The effects of CB clothing and equipment on U.S. Army soldiers' performance: a critical assessment of performance testing. Technical Memorandum 25-80. Aberdeen Proving Ground, Md.: U.S. Army Human Engineering Laboratory.

CBIAC (Chemical and Biological Defense Information and Analysis Center). 1999. Technologies Table on Oxidizing Decontamination in the CB Decontamination Database CD-ROM, Release One. Aberdeen Proving Ground, Md.: CBIAC.

Chairman of the Joint Chiefs of Staff. 1997. Requirements Generation System (Formerly MOP 77). CJCSI 3170.01. Washington, D.C.: Chairman of the Joint Chiefs of Staff.

Chang. M. 1984. A Survey and Evaluation of Chemical Warfare Agent Contaminants and Decontamination. AD-202525. Dugway, Utah: U.S. Army Dugway Proving Ground.

Cheng, T., J.J. Defrank, M.N. Miller, D.K. Vervier, and H.S. Heitz. 1991. Immunochemical and Nucleic Acid Screening of Bacteria for Organophosphate-Degrading Enzymes. Pp. 763–771 in Proceedings of the 1991 U.S. Army Edgewood Research, Development, and Engineering Center Scientific Conference on Chemical Defense Research. Aberdeen Proving Ground, Md.: Edgewood Research, Development, and Engineering Center.

Chow, B.G., G.S. Jones, I. Lachow, J. Stillon, S. Wilkening, and H. Yee. 1998. Air Force Operations in a Chemical and Biological Environment. Rand Report DB-189/1-AF. Santa Monica, Calif.: Rand.

Chue, K.T., J.N. Kim, Y.J. Yoo, S.H. Cho, and R.T. Yang. 1995. Comparison of Activated Carbon and Zeolite 13X for CO_2 Recovery from Flu Gas by Pressure Swing Absorption. Industrial Engineering Chemical Research 34(2): 591–598.

Commission to Assess the Organization of the Federal Government to Combat the Proliferation of Weapons of Mass Destruction. 1999. Combating Proliferation of Weapons of Mass Destruction. Washington, D.C.: Commission to Assess the Organization of the Federal Government to Combat the Proliferation of Weapons of Mass Destruction.

Committee on Veterans' Affairs. 1998. Report of the Special Investigation Unit on Gulf War Illnesses, One Hundred Fifth Congress. Washington, D.C.: U.S. Government Printing Office.

Coombes, R.A., B. Hampson, and J.A.W. Sykes. 1994. A Pressure and Temperature Swing Absorption Filtration System for the Removal of Organic Vapors from an Air Stream. Pp. 561–571 in 1993 Edgewood Research, Development, and Engineering Center Scientific Conference on Chemical Defense Research. Aberdeen Proving Ground, Md.: Edgewood Research, Development, and Engineering Center.

Courtney, R.C., R.L. Gustafson, S.J. Westerback, H. Hyytiainen, S.C. Chaberek, and A.E. Martell. 1957. Metal chelate compounds as catalysts in the hydrolysis of isopropyl methylphosphonofluoridate and diisopropyl phosphorofluoridate. Journal of the American Chemical Society 79: 3030–3036.

Currier, R. 1999. Decontamination using fenton-related reagents and gases. Presentation to the 1999 Department of Energy Chemical and Biological Nonproliferation Program Summer Meeting, McLean, Virginia, July 22, 1999.

Davis, W. 1998. Masks/Development and Production. Presentation by W. Davis, Program Manager, Soldier and Biological Chemical Command, to principal investigators and members of the Advisory Panel on Strategies to Protect the Health of Deployed U.S. Forces, Task 2.3: Physical Protection and Decontamination, Soldier and Biological Chemical Command, Edgewood, Maryland, October 13, 1998.

Day, S.E. 1996. DS2: Development, Improvements, and Replacements. ERDEC-TR-263. Aberdeen Proving Ground, Md.: Edgewood Research, Development, and Engineering Center.

DoD. 1995. Counterproliferation Program Review Committee Report on Activities and Programs for Countering Proliferation. Washington, D.C.: Counterproliferation Program Review Committee.

DoD. 1996. Proliferation: Threat and Response. Washington, D.C.: U.S. Government Printing Office.

DoD. 1997a. Counterproliferation Program Review Committee CPRC Annual Report. Washington, D.C.: U.S. Department of Defense.

DoD. 1997b. Mission-Oriented Protective Posture (MOPP) and Chemical Protection. Information Paper. Washington, D.C.: Special Assistant for Gulf War Illnesses, U.S. Department of Defense.

DoD 1998a. Unit Chemical and Biological Defense Readiness Training. Audit Report. Washington, D.C.: U.S. Department of Defense Inspector General.

DoD. 1998b. Nuclear/Biological/Chemical (NBC) Defense. Annual Report to Congress. Washington, D.C.: U.S. Department of Defense.

DoD. 1999. Nuclear/Biological/Chemical (NBC) Defense. Annual Report to Congress. Washington, D.C.: U.S. Department of Defense.

Dominguez, D.D., R.A. McGill, and R. Chung. 1998. Development of a Carbon Bed Monitor Using a SAW Chemical Sensor. Pp. 477–485 in Proceedings of the 1997 Edgewood Research, Development, and Engineering Center Scientific Conference on Chemical Defense Research. Aberdeen Proving Ground, Md.: Edgewood Research, Development, and Engineering Center.

Draper, E.S., and J.J. Lombardi. 1986. Combined arms in a nuclear/chemical environment force development testing and experimentation, CANE FDTE Summary Evaluation Report, Phase I. Fort McClellan, Ala.: U.S. Army Chemical School.

Eck, B. 1998. General Military Intelligence Aspects of Chemical Warfare. Presentation by B. Eck, Defense Intelligence Agency, to principal investigators of the Strategies to Protect the Health of Deployed U.S. Forces, Task 2.3: Physical Protection and Decontamination. National Research Council, Washington, D.C., June 29, 1998.

Elsner, P., E. Berardesca, and H.I. Maibach. 1994. Bioengineering of the Skin: Water and the Stratum Corneum. Boca Raton, Fla.: CRC Press.

Epstein, J., V.E. Bauer, M. Saxe, and M.M. Demek. 1956. Chlorine-catalyzed hydrolysis of isopropyl methylphosphonoflouridate (sarin) in aqueous solution. Journal of the American Chemical Society 78: 4068–4071.

Fadem, M.E., and C-C.Tsai. 1998. Multi-Stage Bioaerosol Filtration System. Pp. 441–445 in Proceedings of the 1997 Edgewood Research, Development, and Engineering Center Scientific Conference on Chemical Defense Research. Aberdeen Proving Ground, Md.: Edgewood Research, Development, and Engineering Center.

Ford, M.S., and W.E. Newton. 1989. International Materiel Evaluation of the German C8 Emulsion. DPG-FR-88-009. Dugway, Utah: U.S. Army Dugway Proving Ground.

Friel, J.V., and M.G. Graham. 1989. Sacrificial Coatings Agent Evaluation. NATICK/TR-91/042. Pittsburgh, Pa.: MSA Research Corporation.

Frosch, P.J., A. Kurte, and B. Pilz. 1993a. Biophysical Techniques for the Evaluation of Skin Protective Creams. Pp. 214–222 in Noninvasive Methods for the Quantification of Skin Functions, P.J. Frosch and A.M. Kligman, eds. Berlin: Springer-Verlag.

Frosch, P.J., A. Kurte, and B. Pilz. 1993b. Efficacy of skin barrier creams. 3. The repetitive irritation test (RIT) in humans. Contact Dermatitis 29: 113–118.

Frosch, P.J., A. Schulze-Dirks, M. Hoffmann, and I. Axthelm. 1993c. Efficacy of skin barrier creams. 2. Ineffectiveness of a popular "skin protector" against various irritants in the repetitive irritation test in the guinea pig. Contact Dermatitis 29: 74–77.

Frosch, P.J., A. Schulze-Dirks, M. Hoffmann, I. Axthelm, and A. Kurte. 1993d. Efficacy of skin barrier creams. 1. The repetitive irritation test (RIT) in the guinea pig. Contact Dermatitis 28: 94–100.

Frosch, P.J., and A. Kurte. 1994. Efficacy of skin barrier creams. 4. The repetitive irritation test (RIT) with a set of four standard irritants. Contact Dermatitis 31: 161–168.

Fullerton, A., and T. Menne. 1995. In vitro and in vivo evaluation of the effect of barrier gels in nickel contact allergy. Contact Dermatitis 32: 100–106.

Gander, T.J. 1997. Jane's NBC Protection Equipment, 10th ed. Surrey, U.K.: Jane's Information Group, Inc.

GAO. 1999. Combating Terrorism: Observations on the Nunn-Lugar-Dominici Domestic Preparedness Program. Audit Report. Washington, D.C.: General Accounting Office.

Garrison, J.M., D.R. Knudsen, and W.M. Waskom. 1982. Shipboard chemical warfare training exercise. NSWC TR 82-431. Dahlgren, Va.: Naval Surface Weapons Center.

Gawron, V., H. Taylor, J. Howe, R. Hughes, D. Stevens, T. Swalm, D. Hilmas, and R. Fuchs. 1998. Report on United States Air Force Expeditionary Forces. Vol. 3, App. I. Washington, D.C.: U.S. Air Force.

Gibson, H., and D. Reneker. 1998. Nanofibers: New Fabric Architectures. Presentation to the U.S. Army Nanotechnology Conference, Boston, Massachusetts, July 7–9, 1998.

Gibson, P.W. and H. Schreuder-Gibson. 1999. Aerosol Particle Filtration, Gas Flow, and Vapor Diffusion Properties of Electrospun Nanofiber Coatings. Natick/TR-99/016L. Natick, Mass.: U.S. Army Soldier and Biological Chemical Command.

Gibson, P.W., H.L. Schreuder-Gibson, and D. Rivin. 1999. Electrospun fiber mats: transport properties. American Institute of Chemical Engineers Journal 45(1): 190–194.

Goh, C.L. 1991a. Cutting oil dermatitis on guinea pig skin. 1. Cutting oil dermatitis and barrier cream. Contact Dermatitis 24: 16–21.

Goh, C.L. 1991b. Cutting oil dermatitis on guinea pig skin. 2. Emollient creams and cutting oil dermatitis. Contact Dermatitis 24: 81–85.

Goh, C.L., and S.L. Gan. 1994. Efficacies of a barrier cream and an afterwork emollient cream against cutting fluid dermatitis in metalworkers: a prospective study. Contact Dermatitis 31: 176–180.

Goldman, R.F., and the Staff of the Military Ergonomics Division, United States Army Research Institute of Environmental Medicine. 1981. CW protective clothing: the nature of its performance degradation and some partial solutions. Natick, Mass.: United States Army Research Institute of Environmental Medicine.

Gray, K.A., and R.J. Hilarides. 1995. Radiolytic treatment of dioxin contaminated soils. Radiation Physical Chemistry 46: 1081–1084.

Grevelink, S.A., D.F. Murrell, and E.A. Olsen. 1992. Effectiveness of various barrier preparations in preventing and/or ameliorating experimentally produced toxicodendron dermatitis. Journal of the American Academy of Dermatology 27: 182–188.

Grunewald, A. M., J. Lorenz, M. Gloor, W. Gehring, and P. Kleesz. 1996. Lipophilic irritants: protective value of urea- and of glycerol-containing oil-in-water emulsions. Dermatosen in Beruf und Umwelt 44: 81–86.

REFERENCES

Gupta, S.K., E.D. Bashaw, and S.S. Hwang. 1993. Pharmacokinetic and Pharmacodynamic Modeling of Transdermal Products. Pp. 311–330 in Topical Drug Bioavailability, Bioequivalence, and Penetration, V.P. Shah and H.I. Maibach eds. New York: Plenum Press.

Harvey, S.P., W.T. Beaudry, P.C. Bossle, J.E. Kolakowski, L.R. Procell, D.K. Rohrbaugh, D.C. Sorrick, A.N. Stroup, L.L. Szafraniec, Y.C. Yang, and G.W. Wagner. 1997. Caustic Hydrolysis of Sulfur Mustard. ERDEC-TR-385. Aberdeen Proving Ground, Md.: Edgewood Research, Development, and Engineering Center.

Henderson, V.D., and T.J. Novak. 1992. Vapor-Pulse, Filter-Life Indicator Concept Incorporating a Liquid Crystal. CRDEC-TR-403. Aberdeen Proving Ground, Md.: U.S. Army.

Hermansky, C., and R.A. Mackay. 1979. Reactions in Microemulsions: Phosphate Ester Hydrolysis. Pp. 723–730 in Solution Chemistry of Surfactants. New York: Plenum Press.

Hinds, W.C. 1999. Respiratory Protection. Presentation by W.C. Hinds, University of California School of Public Health, to principal investigators and members of the Advisory Panel on Strategies to Protect the Health of Deployed U.S. Forces, Task 2.3: Physical Protection and Decontamination, National Research Council, Washington, D.C., January 25, 1999.

Hurst, C.G. 1997. Decontamination. Pp. 351–359 in Textbook of Military Medicine, Medical Aspects of Chemical and Biological Warfare. Washington, D.C.: Walter Reed Army Medical Center.

Institute for Defense Analyses. 1999. Informal briefing to principal investigators and the National Research Council staff, Institute for Defense Analyses, Alexandria, Virginia, April 6, 1999.

IOM (Institute of Medicine). 1999a. Strategies to Protect Deployed Forces: Medical Surveillance, Record Keeping, and Risk Reduction. Medical Follow-up Agency. Washington, D.C.: National Academy Press.

IOM. 1999b. Chemical and Biological Terrorism Research and Development to Improve Civilian Medical Response. Committee on R&D Needs for Improving Civilian Medical Response to Chemical and Biological Terrorism Incidents. Washington, D.C.: National Academy Press.

Irving, P.M. 1998. Portable plasma flare for surface decontamination. Paper presented at the Scientific Conference on Chemical and Biological Defense Research, Edgewood Research, Development, and Engineering Center, Aberdeen Proving Ground, Maryland, November 18, 1998.

Irving, G., T. McMurray, J. Herbold. 1997. Non-Medical Dispersed Biological Weapons Countermeasures. San Antonio, Texas: Conceptual Mindworks, Inc.

Ito, H., Y. Ohki, Y. Watanabe, H. Sunaga, and I. Ishhigaki. 1993. Sterilization of bacillus spores by converted x-rays. Radiation Physical Chemistry 42(4–6): 597–600.

Jaeger, D.A., J. Wettstein, and A. Zafar. 1998. Cleavable quaternary hydrazinium surfactants. Langmuir 14: 1940–1941.

Johnson, K.M. 1990. Marburg and Ebola Viruses. Pp. 1303–1306 in Principles and Practice of Infectious Disease, 3rd Ed. New York: Churchill Livingstone.

Joint Chiefs of Staff. 1995. Joint Doctrine for Nuclear, Biological, and Chemical (NBC) Defense. Joint Publication 3-11, July 10, 1995. Washington, D.C.: Joint Chiefs of Staff.

Joint Chiefs of Staff. 1996. Joint Vision 2010. Washington, D.C.: Joint Chiefs of Staff.

Joint Chiefs of Staff. 1998. Deployment Health Surveillance and Readiness. Memorandum to Under Secretary of Defense for Personnel and Readiness, December 4, 1998.

Joint Science and Technology Panel for CB Defense. 1999. Joint Science and Technology Chemical and Biological Decontamination Master Plan Summary. Washington, D.C.: U.S. Department of Defense.

Joseph, R.G. 1996. The impact of NBC proliferation on doctrine and operations. Joint Force Quarterly 13: 74–80.

Katz, S.A. 1990. Chemical Speciation and Bioavailability of Chromium from ASC Carbon. CRDEC-CR-088. Aberdeen Proving Ground, Md.: U.S. Army.

Katz, S.A. 1999. Contaminant Air Removal. Presentation by S.A. Katz, Rutgers University, to principal investigators and members of the Advisory Panel on Strategies to Protect the Health of Deployed U.S. Forces, Task 2.3: Physical Protection and Decontamination, National Research Council, Washington, D.C., January 25, 1999.

Kelly, T.L., C.E. Englund, D.H. Ryman, J.E. Yeager, and A.A. Sucec. 1988. The effects of 12 hours of MOPP IV gear on cognitive performance under nonexcercise conditions. San Diego, Calif.: Naval Health Research Center.

Kerch, J. 1998. M291 and M295 Decontamination Kit. Presentation by J. Kerch to the Decontamination Commodity Area Program Review Meeting, Joint Service Materiel Group, Edgewood, Maryland, October 7–8, 1998.

Kirkwood, C. 1998. Mask Protection: From Threat to Requirement. Presentation by C. Kirkwood, U.S. Army Chemical School, to principal investigators and members of the Advisory Panel on Strategies to Protect the Health of Deployed U.S. Forces, Task 2.3: Physical Protection and Decontamination, Ft. McClellan, Alabama, August 11, 1998.

Ko, F.K. 1999. Textile and Garments. Presentation by F.K. Ko, Drexel University, to principal investigators and members of the Advisory Panel on Strategies to Protect the Health of Deployed U.S. Forces, Task 2.3: Physical Protection and Decontamination. National Research Council, Washington, D.C., January 26, 1999.

Ko, F.K., C.T. Laurencin, M.D. Borden, and D. Reneker. 1998. Dynamics of Cell Fiber Architecture Interaction. Pp. 11 in Proceedings of the Biomaterials Research Society Annual Meeting. San Diego, Calif.: Society of Biomaterials.

Kolakowski, J.E., J.J. DeFrank, S.P. Harvey, L.L. Szafraniec, W.T. Beaudry, and W. Laikh. 1997. Enzymatic hydrolysis of the chemical warfare agent-VX and its neurotoxic analogs by organophosphorous hydrolase. Biocatalysis and Biotransformation 15: 297–312.

Kuhlmann, W.D. 1998. Respiratory Protection. Presentation by W. Kuhlmann, Team Leader, Respiratory and Collective Protection Team R&T Directorate, Soldier and Biological Chemical Command, to principal investigators and members of the Advisory Panel on Strategies to Protect the Health of Deployed U.S. Forces, Task 2.3: Physical Protection and Decontamination, Soldier and Biological Chemical Command, Edgewood, Maryland, October 13, 1998.

Lai, K., K.I. Dave, J.R. Wild, L.L. Szafraniec, W.T. Beaudry, S.P. Harvey. 1994. Enzymatic Decontamination of Organophosphorus Chemical Agents by Genetic and Biochemical Manipulation of Organophosphorus Hydrolase. Pp. 887–893 in Proceedings of the 1993 Edgewood Research, Development, and Engineering Center Scientific Conference on Chemical Defense Research. Aberdeen Proving Ground, Md.: Edgewood Research, Development, and Engineering Center.

Landsberg, M.I. 1964. Collective Protection for Combat Field Structures. LSI-2651. Saint Paul, Minn.: Litton Systems, Inc.

LeDuc, J.W. 1989. Epidemiology of hemorrhagic fever viruses. Reviews of Infectious Diseases 11(Supp. 4): S730–S725.

LeJeune, K.E., B.C. Dravis, F.Yang, A.D. Hetro, B.P. Doctor, and A.J. Russell. 1998. Fighting nerve agent chemical weapons with enzyme technology. Annals of the New York Academy of Sciences 864: 153–170.

LeJeune, K.E., and A.J. Russell. 1999. Biocatalytic nerve agent detoxification in fire fighting foams. Biotechnology and Bioengineering 62(6): 659–665.

Leslie, D.R., W.T. Beaudry, and L.L. Szafraniec. 1991. Sorption and Reaction of Chemical Agents by a Mixed Sorptive/Reactive Resin. CRDEC-TR-292. Aberdeen Proving Ground, Md.: U.S. Army.

Letts, K., and R.A. Mackay. 1975. Reactions in microemulsions. 1. Metal-ion incorporation by tetraphenylporphine. Inorganic Chemistry 14: 2990–2993.

Leung, H.W., and D.J. Paustenbach. 1994. Techniques for estimating the percutaneous absorption of chemicals due to occupational and environmental exposure. Applied Occupational and Environmental Hygiene 9: 187–197.

Lielke, M., T.C. McDonald, T.W. Mix, and R.P. Northey. 1986. Colorimetric Concepts for Residual Filter Life Indicator. CRDEC-CR-86028. Aberdeen Proving Ground, Md.: U.S. Army.

Longchamp, P. 1999. Evolution of Industrial Enzymes by DNA Shuffling for Decontamination of Biological and Chemical Warfare Agents. Paper presented at the 1999 Joint Chemical and Biological Decontamination Conference, Joint Service Materiel Group. Nashville, Tennessee, June 8–10, 1999.

Mahmoud, G., and J.M. Lachapelle. 1985. Evaluation of the protective value of an antisolvent gel by laser Doppler flowmetry and histology. Contact Dermatitis 13: 14–19.

Marks, J.G., Jr., J.F. Fowler, E.F. Sherertz, and R.L. Rietschel. 1995. Prevention of poison ivy and poison oak allergic contact dermatitis by quaternium-18 bentonite. Journal of the American Academy of Dermatology 33: 212–216.

Marzulli, F.N., and H.I. Maibach. 1991. Dermatotoxicology. New York: Hemisphere Publishing.

McClain, D.C., and F.J. Storrs. 1992. Protective effect of both a barrier cream and a polyethylene laminate glove against epoxy resin, glyceryl monothioglycolate, frullania, and tansy. American Journal of Contact Dermatitis 3: 201–205.

McDougal, J.N. 1991. Physiologically Based Pharmacokinetic Modeling. Pp. 37–60 in Dermatotoxicology, 4th ed. F.N. Marzulli and H.I. Maibach, eds. New York: Hemisphere Publishing.

McDougal, J.N. 1998. Methods in Physiologically Based Pharmacokinetic Modeling. Pp.51–68 in Dermatotoxicology Methods: The Laboratory Worker's Vade Mecum. F.N. Marzulli and H.I. Maibach, eds. Washington, D.C.: Taylor & Francis.

McGuire, R., D. Shepley, D.M. Hoffman, A. Alcaraz, and E. Raber. 1999. Oxidative Decontamination. Paper presented at the 1999 Joint Chemical and Biological Decontamination Conference, Joint Service Materiel Group. Nashville, Tennessee, June 8–10, 1999.

McKnight, D., M. O'Dell, W. Cooper, G. Knudson, and G. Loda. 1999. Surebeam™ Decon, A Versatile Technology for the Battlefield. Paper presented at the 1999 Joint Service Chemical Biological Decontamination Conference, Joint Service Materiel Group. Nashville, Tennessee, June 8–10, 1999.

Medema, J. 1999. Proposed NATO Long-Term Scientific Study (LTSS) Chemical and Biological Defense. Paper presented to the 1999 Joint Service Chemical Biological Decontamination Conference, Joint Service Materiel Group. Nashville, Tennessee, June 8–10, 1999.

Medema J., J.J.G.M. Van Bokhoven, and A.E.T. Kuiper. 1987. The Design of a Self-Decontaminating Adsorbent. Rijswijk, Netherlands: TNO Prins Maurits Laboratorium.

Mellian, S.A. 1997. Final Phase II Design, Size and Fit Evaluation Report. Report M67854-95-C-1028. Natick, Mass.: U.S. Navy Clothing and Textile Research Facility.

Mellian, S.A. 1999. Design and Sizing System Development: JSLIST, Gloves, Boots. Presentation by S.A. Mellian, Navy Clothing and Textile Research Facility, to principal investigators and members of the Advisory Panel on Strategies to Protect the Health of Deployed U.S. Forces, Task 2.3: Physical Protection and Decontamination, National Research Council, Washington, D.C., January 25, 1999.

Menger, F.M., L.H. Gan, E. Johnson, and D.H. Durst. 1987. Phosphate ester hydrolysis catalyzed by metallomicelles. Journal of the American Chemical Society 109(9): 2800–2803.

Menger, F.M., and A.R. Elrington. 1991. Organic reactivity in microemulsion system. Journal of the American Chemical Society 113: 9621–9724.

Menger, F.M., and H. Park. 1994. Microemulsions as reaction media: self-organizing assemblies in an environmental cleanup problem. Recueil des Travaux Chimiques de Pays-Bas 113: 176–180.

Mikolajczyk, M. 1989. Scientific Advances in Alternative Demilitarization Technologies. Boston, Mass.: Kluwer Academic Publishers.

Mikolich, D.J., and J.M. Boyce. 1990. Brucella Species. Pp. 1735–1742 in Principles and Practice of Infectious Disease, 3rd ed. New York: Churchill Livingstone.

Morrison, R. 1998. Advanced Adsorbents for Protection. Presentation by R. Morrison, Soldier and Biological Chemical Command, to principal investigators and members of the Advisory Panel on Strategies to Protect the Health of Deployed U.S. Forces, Task 2.3: Physical Protection and Decontamination. Soldier and Biological Chemical Command, Edgewood, Maryland, October 13, 1998.

Moss, R.A., K.W. Alwis, and G.O. Bizzigotti. 1983. Ortho-iodosobenzoate: catalyst for the micellar cleavage of activated esters and phosphates. Journal of the American Chemical Society 105: 681–682.

Moss, R.A., K.Y. Kim, and S. Swarup. 1986. Efficient catalytic cleavage of reactive phosphates by an o-iodosobenzoate functionalized surfactant. Journal of the American Chemical Society 108: 788–793.

Moss, R.A., and H. Zhang. 1993. Toward a broad spectrum decontaminant for reactive toxic phosphates/phosphonates: n-alkyl-3-iodosopyridinium-4-carboxylates. Tetrahedron Letters 34: 6225–6228.

NATO (North Atlantic Treaty Organization). 1996a. NATO Handbook on the Medical Aspects of NBC Defense Operations. Part III Chemical. AMedP-6(B). Washington, D.C.: U.S. Government Printing Office.

NATO. 1996b. NATO Handbook on the Medical Aspects of NBC Defense Operations. Part II Biological. AMedP-6(B). Washington, D.C.: U.S. Government Printing Office.

Negron, A. 1998. Advanced Integrated Collective Protection System. Presentation by A. Negron. Soldier and Biological Chemical Command, to principal investigators and members of the Advisory Panel on Strategies to Protect the Health of Deployed U.S. Forces, Task 2.3: Physical Protection and Decontamination. Soldier and Biological Chemical Command, Edgewood, Maryland, October 13, 1998.

Nene, D.M., R.M. Kopchik, W.H. Brendley, M.A. Koals, and V.M. McHugh. 1988. Composition, Formulation Method, Test Development, and Performance Evaluation Investigations of Sorptive/Catalytic Self-Decontaminating Coatings. Philadelphia, Pa.: Rohm and Haas Company.

Nieuwenhuizen, M.S., J.L. Harteveld, R.C. Oliver, and E.R. Wils. 1998. Development of a Filter Life Indicator System (FLIS). PML-1997-A104. Rijswijk, Netherlands: TNO Prins Maurits Laboratorium.

Nilo, P. 1999. Service Integration: JSIG/JSMG Process. Presentation by P. Nilo, U.S. Army, to principal investigators and members of the Advisory Panel on Strategies to Protect the Health of Deployed U.S. Forces, Task 2.3: Physical Protection and Decontamination, National Research Council, Washington, D.C., January 25, 1999.

NRC (National Research Council). 1985. Possible Long-Term Health Effects of Short-Term Exposure To Chemical Agents. Vol. 3, Final Report. Board on Toxicology and Environmental Health Hazards. Washington, D.C.: National Academy Press.

NRC. 1997a. Review of Acute Human-Toxicity Estimates for Selected Chemical-Warfare Agents. Committee on Toxicology. Washington, D.C.: National Academy Press.

NRC. 1997b. Technical Assessment of the Man-In-Simulant Test (MIST) Program. Board on Army Science and Technology. Washington, D.C.: National Academy Press.

NRC. 1999a. Technology-Based Pilot Programs. Commission on Engineering and Technical Systems. Washington, D.C.: National Academy Press.

NRC. 1999b. Strategies to Protect Deployed U.S. Forces: Detecting, Characterizing, and Documenting Exposures. Division of Military Science and Technology, Commission on Engineering and Technical Systems. Washington, D.C.: National Academy Press.

NRC. 1999c. Strategies to Protect Deployed U.S. Forces: Risk Assessment. Board on Environmental Studies and Toxicology, Commission on Life Sciences. Washington, D.C.: National Academy Press.

NRC. 1999d. Discussion at the Workshop on Strategies to Protect the Health of Deployed U.S. Forces, Task 2.3: Physical Protection and Decontamination, National Research Council, Washington, D.C., January 25–26, 1999.

NRC. 1999e. Review of Acute Human-Toxicity Estimates for Selected Chemical-Warfare Agents. Subcommittee on Chronic Reference Doses for Selected Chemical Warfare Agents. Washington, D.C.: National Academy Press.

Olivarius, F. D. F., A.B. Hansen, T. Karlsmark, and H.C. Wulf. 1996. Water protective effect of barrier creams and moisturizing creams: a new in-vivo test method. Contact Dermatitis 35: 219–225.

Packham, C.L., H.L. Packham, and R. Russell-Fell. 1994. Evaluation of barrier creams: an in vitro technique on human skin. Acta Dermatologica Venereolica 74: 405–406.

Payne, J. 1998. Chemical Vision 2010. Presentation by J. Payne, U.S. Army Chemical School, to principal investigators and members of the Advisory Panel on Strategies to Protect the Health of Deployed U.S. Forces, Task 2.3: Physical Protection and Decontamination. U.S. Army Chemical School, Ft. McClellan, Alabama, August 11, 1998.

Persian Gulf Veterans Coordinating Board. 1997. The Persian Gulf Veterans Coordinating Board Action Plan with Respect to the Findings and Recommendations of the Presidential Advisory Committee on Gulf War Veteran's Illnesses Final Report. Washington, D.C.: U.S. Department of Defense.

Price, C.C., and O.H. Bullitt. 1943. The Chemistry of Mustard Gas as a Water Contaminant. Edgewood Arsenal, Md.: CWS Technical Command Chemical Warfare Center.

Raber, E., R. McGuire, D. Shepley, M. Hoffman, A. Alcarez, W. Earl, and R. Currier. 1998. Oxidizers: The Solution for Chemical Agent Decontamination. Paper presented at the Department of Energy Chemical and Biological Nonproliferation Program, McLean, Virginia, July 29, 1998.

Raines, S. 1999. Pope/Bragg Study. Paper presented at the 1999 Joint Service Chemical Biological Decontamination Conference, Joint Service Materiel Group, Nashville, Tennessee, June 8–10, 1999.

Rakaczky, J.A. 1981. The effect of chemical protective clothing and equipment on combat efficiency. Technical Report #313. Aberdeen Proving Ground, Md.: U.S. Army Material Systems Analysis Activity.

Reneker, D.H., and I. Chun. 1996. Nanometer diameter fibers of polymer produced by electrospinning. Nanotechnology 7: 216–223.

Renneke, R.F. 1998. NO_x Absorber for CATOX/ECU System. Pp. 487–493 in 1997 Edgewood Research, Development, and Engineering Center Scientific Conference on Chemical Defense Research. Aberdeen Proving Ground, Md.: Edgewood Research, Development, and Engineering Center.

Reuter, J.D. 1998. Inhibition of Influenza Virus Infection in Mice Using Intranasal Liposome-like Nanoemulsions. Presention by J.D. Reuter to the 38th Interscience Conference on Antimicrobial Agents and Chemotherapy, American Society for Microbiology. San Diego, California, September 24–27, 1998.

Rhodes, J.E., H.L. Cowan, A.L. Skarzenski, J. Williams, and P. Coon. 1998. Proceedings of the 9th International Simulant Workshop. ERDEC-SP-057. Aberdeen Proving Ground, Md.: Edgewood Research, Development, and Engineering Center, U.S. Army Chemical and Biological Defense Command.

Rhodes, J.E., and M. Decker. 1999. Unconventional Threats. Available on-line at: http://www.house.gov/hasc/testimony/106thcongress/99-02-11rhodes-decker.htm.

Rhule, J.T., R.P. Johnson, and C.L. Hill. 1998a. New Polyoxymetalate-TSPs for CW Agent Detection and Decontamination. Paper presented at the Scientific Conference on Chemical and Biological Defense Research, Edgewood Research, Development, and Engineering Center, Aberdeen Proving Ground, Md., November 20, 1998.

Rhule, J.T., C.L. Hill, and D.A. Judd. 1998b. Polyoxymetallates in medicine. Chemical Reviews 98(1): 327–357.

Richardson, D.E., R.S. Drago, K.M. Frank, G.W. Wagner, and Y.C. Yang. 1998. Kinetics and Equilibrium Formation of Weakly Basic Oxidant System for Decontamination. Paper presented at the Scientific Conference on Chemical and Biological Defense Research, Edgewood Research, Development, and Engineering Center, Aberdeen Proving Ground, Maryland, November 20, 1998.

Richardson, G.A. 1972. Development of Package Decontaminating System. EACR-1310-17, Final Report. DAAA15-71-C-0508. Dayton, Ohio: Monsanto Research Corporation.

Richmond, J.A., A.B. Livesey, D. Fielder, and W.C. Johnson.1990. Removal of nuclear, chemical and biological contaminants from electronics. Pp. 779–805 in Proceedings of the Tactical Communications Conference. Vol.1. Tactical Communications Challenges of the 1990s. New York: IEEE.

Rose, J.B. In press. Future Health Assessment and Risk Management Integration for Infectious Diseases and Biological Weapons for Deployed United States Forces. Workshop Proceedings of the Strategies to Protect the Health of Deployed U.S. Forces: Assessing Health Risks to Deployed U.S. Forces. Washington, D.C.: National Academy Press.

Rossin, J.A. 1996. Catalytic Reactor System Concepts for Military Air Purification Applications. CRDEC-CR-221. Aberdeen Proving Ground, Md.: U.S. Army.

Roth, R. 1982. Current Status of Research, Development, and Testing of Fabrics for Chemical/Biological Warfare. Presentation by R. Roth to the Outlook '82 Industrial Fabrics Association International 23rd Conference, New York, May 19, 1982.

Russell, A.J., and K.E. LeJeune. 1999. Utilizing the enzyme catalysis in the decontamination and detection of nerve agent chemical weapons. Paper presented at the 1999 Joint Chemical and Biological Decontamination Conference, Joint Service Materiel Group, Nashville, Tennessee, June 8, 1999.

Sagripanti, J.L., and A. Bonifacino. 1996. Comparative sporicidal effects of liquid chemical agents. Applied and Environmental Microbiology 62: 545–551.

Schilling, C.L., B. Li, E. Kubiczloring, and D.A. Jaeger. 1997. Characterization of a vesicular dithiophosphate surfactant and its application in chemical agent decontamination. Abstracts of the American Chemical Society 214(2): 252.

SchlÅter-Wigger, W., and P. Elsner. 1996. Efficacy of four commercially available protective creams in the repetitive irritation test (RIT). Contact Dermatitis 34: 278–283.

Schreuder-Gibson, H. 1998. Electrospinlacing. Presentation by H. Schreuder-Gibson, Soldier and Biological Chemical Command to principal investigators and members of the Advisory Panel on Strategies to Protect the Health of Deployed U.S. Forces, Task 2.3: Physical Protection and Decontamination, Soldier and Biological Chemical Command, Soldier Systems Center, Natick, Massachusetts, November 16, 1998.

Secretary of Defense. 1999. Annual Report to the President and the Congress. Washington, D.C.: Office of the Secretary of Defense.

Selwyn, D., and R. Currier. 1999. Personal communication between D. Selwyn, R. Currier, Los Alamos National Laboratory, and Maher Tadros, Sandia National Laboratories.

Shah, V.P., G.L. Flynn, R.H. Guy, H.I. Maibach, H. Schaefer, J.P. Skelly, R.C. Wester, and A. Yacobi. 1991. In vivo percutaneous penetration/absorption. Pharmacological Research 8: 1071–1075.

Shah, V.P., D. Hare, S.V. Dighe, and R.L. Williams. 1993. Bioequivalence of Topical Dermatological Products. Pp. 393–412 in Topical Drug Bioavailability, Bioequivalence, and Penetration, V.P. Shah and H.I. Maibach, eds. New York: Plenum Press.

Shipton, D.L., K.R. Beilstein, A.P. Chenzoff, R.L Pitzer, and R.P. Joyce. 1988. Effects of chemical warfare defense on airbase maintenance operations, Phase II report. AFHRL-TR-87-32. Wright-Patterson Air Force Base, Ohio: Air Force Human Resources Laboratory.

Siegel, J. 1998. Collective Protection. Presentation by J. Siegel, U.S. Army Soldier and Biological Chemical Command (SBCCOM), Soldier Center of Excellence (SCOE), to principal investigators and members of the Advisory Panel Members on Strategies to Protect the Health of Deployed U.S. Forces, Task 2.3: Physical Protection and Decontamination, Soldier and Biological Chemical Command, Natick, Massachusetts, November 16, 1998.

Stallings, R.L. 1984. Collective Protection by Pressure Swing Adsorption. Paper presented at 1984 Scientific Conference on Chemical Defense Research, Edgewood Research, Development, and Engineering Center, Aberdeen Proving Ground, Maryland, November 13–16, 1984.

Stevens, J.I., and V. Henderson. 1987. Self-Decontaminating Coatings. Pp. 965–968 in Proceedings of the U.S. Army Chemical Research, Development and Engineering Center Scientific Conference on Chemical Defense Research. Aberdeen, Md.: Edgewood Research, Development, and Engineering Center.

Tadros, M.E. 1999. Decontamination Technologies. Presentation by M.E. Tadros, Sandia National Laboratories, to principal investigators and members of the Advisory Panel on Strategies to Protect the Health of Deployed U.S. Forces, Task 2.3: Physical Protection and Decontamination. National Research Council, Washington, D.C., January 25, 1999.

Tadros, M.E., K. Bridger, A. Berrier, R. Hearns, and D. Woodbury. 1986. Enhanced hydrolysis of diphenyl chlorophosphate and agent GD by tetrapentyl ammonium bromide. Paper presented at the Scientific Conference on Chemical and Biological Defense Research, Edgewood Research, Development, and Engineering Center, Aberdeen Proving Ground, Maryland, November 18-21, 1986.

Tadros, M.E., M.D. Tucker, and J.G. Teterycz. 1998. Aqueous Foam for Mitigation and Decontamination of Chemical and Biological Weapons Agents. Paper presented at the Scientific Conference on Chemical and Biological Defense Research, Edgewood Research, Development, and Engineering Center, Aberdeen Proving Ground, Maryland, November 20, 1998.

Talamo, E., G. Meyer, M. Diederen, and M. Pence. 1994. DS2 Reformulation and Packaging Study. ERDEC-CR-120. Aberdeen Proving Ground, Md.: Edgewood Research, Development, and Engineering Center.

Taylor, H., and J. Orlansky. 1987. The Effects on Human Performance Due to Wearing Protective Clothing for Chemical Warfare: Implications for Training. P2026. Alexandria, Va.: Institute for Defense Analyses.

Taylor, H., and J. Orlansky. 1991. The Effects of Wearing Protective Chemical Warfare Combat Clothing on Human Performance. P2433. Alexandria, Va.: Institute for Defense Analyses.

Taylor, H., and J. Orlansky. 1993. The effects of wearing protective chemical warfare clothing on human performance. Aviation, Space, and Environmental Medicine 64(3): A1–A41.

Treffel, P., B. Gabard, and R. Juch. 1994. Evaluation of barrier creams: an *in vitro* technique on human skin. Acta Dermatologica Venereologica 74: 7–11.

Treffel, P., and B. Gabard. 1996. Bioengineering measurements of barrier creams efficacy against toluene and NaOH in an *in vivo* single irritation test. Skin Research and Technology 2: 83–87.

Tucker, M. D. 1998. Personal communication between M.D. Tucker, Sandia National Laboratories, and Maher Tadros, Sandia National Laboratories, December 21, 1998.

Turman, B.N., S.L. Shope, J.A. Jacobs, M.G. Mazarakis, C.L. Olson, G.M. Loubriel, and J.C. Wehlburg. 1998. Accelerator Technology for Emerging Defense Needs. SAND98-2732. Albuquerque, New Mexico: Sandia National Laboratories.

U.S. Air Force. 1997. USAF Operations in a Chemical and Biological (CB) Warfare Environment, CB Hazards. Air Force Handbook 32-4014, Vol. 2. Washington, D.C.: Department of the Air Force.

U.S. Army. 1986. Phase I: Combined Arms in a Nuclear/Chemical Environment. Summary Evaluation Report. Fort McClellan, Ala.: U.S. Army Chemical School.

U.S. Army. 1987. Assessment of Performance of Tasks by Personnel Dressed in Chemical Protective Clothing. Technical Report, June 1987. Dugway, Utah: Technical Analysis and Information Office, U.S. Army Dugway Proving Ground.

U.S. Army. 1991a. Medical Evacuation in a Theater of Operations: Tactics, Techniques, and Procedures. Army Field Manual FM 8-10-6. Washington, D.C.: Department of the Army.

U.S. Army. 1991b. Acclimatization and Adaptation for Troops in a Mission-Oriented Protective Posture (MOPP). October, 1991. Dugway, Utah: Technical Analysis and Information Office, U.S. Army Dugway Proving Ground.

U.S. Army. 1992. Force Development Test and Experimentation: Combined Arms in a Nuclear/Chemical Environment, Close Combat Light. Test Report, November 1992. Fort Hood, Texas: U.S. Army Test and Experimentation Command.

U.S. Army. 1993. Health Service Support in a Nuclear, Biological, and Chemical Environment. Army Field Manual FM 8-10-7. Washington, D.C.: Department of the Army.

U.S. Army. 1994. Commander's Tactical NBC Handbook. Training Circular 3-1, September, 29, 1994.Washington, D.C.: Headquarters, Department of the Army.

U.S. Army. 1995. Medical Management of Chemical Casualties Handbook. Aberdeen Proving Ground, Md.: Medical Research Institute of Chemical Defense, Chemical Casualty Care Office.

U.S. Army. 1998. Antiterrorism Force Protection (AT/FP): Security of Personnel, Information, and Critical Resources from Asymmetric Attacks. Army Regulation 525-13. Washington, D.C.: U.S. Army.

U.S. Army CHPPM (Center for Health Promotion and Preventive Medicine). 1999. Short Term Chemical Exposure Guidelines for Deployed Military Personnel. USACHPPM TG 230A. Ft. Detrick, Md.: U.S. Army Center for Health Promotion and Preventive Medicine.

U.S. Army Chemical Defense Equipment Process Action Team. 1994. Review of Existing Toxicity Data and Human Estimates for Selected Chemical Agents and Recommended Human Toxicity Estimates Appropriate for Defending the Soldier. Report No. ERDEC-SP-018. Prepared by S.A. Reutter and J.V. Wade. Aberdeen Proving Ground, Md.: U.S. Army Edgewood Research, Development, and Engineering Center.

U.S. Army Medical Research Institute of Infectious Disease. 1998. Medical Management of Biological Casualties Handbook, 3rd ed. Fort Detrick, Frederick, Md.: U.S. Army Medical Research Institute of Infectious Disease.

U.S. Army Office of the Surgeon General. 1997. Textbook of Military Medicine: Medical Aspects of Chemical and Biological Warfare. Washington, D.C.: Walter Reed Army Medical Center.

U.S. Army SBCCOM (Soldier and Biological Chemical Command). 1998. Presentations by employees of SBCCOM Edgewood Chemical and Biological Center, to principal investigators and members of the Advisory Panel of the Study Strategies to Protect the Health of Deployed U.S. Forces, Task 2.3: Physical Protection and Decontamination. Edgewood, Maryland, October 13, 1998.

U.S. Army SBCCOM. 1999. M41 PATS. Available on-line at: http://www.sbccom.apgea.army.mil/RDA/ecbc/engineering/pats.htm.

U.S. Army Soldier Systems Center. 1997. Chemically and Biologically Protected Shelter. Available on-line at: http://www.natick.army.mil/prodprog/sustain/cbps.htm.

U.S. Army Soldier Systems Center. 1999. Joint Transportable Collective Protection System (JTCOPS). Available on-line at: http://www.natick.army.mil/prodprog/sustain/jtcops.htm.

U.S. Army and U.S. Marine Corps. 1992. NBC Protection. Field Manual 3-4 and Fleet Marine Force Manual No. 11-9. Washington, D.C.: Department of the Army and U.S. Marine Corps.

U.S. Army and U.S. Marine Corps. 1993. NBC Decontamination. Army Field Manual 3-5 and Fleet Marine Force Manual No. 11-10. Washington, D.C.: U.S. Army and U.S. Marine Corps.

U.S. Army and U.S. Marine Corps. 1996. Chemical Operations Principles and Fundamentals. Field Manual 3-100 and Marine Corps Warfighting Publication 3-3.7.1. Washington, D.C.: U.S. Army and U.S. Marine Corps.

U.S. Army, U.S. Navy, and U.S. Air Force. 1990. Potential Military Chemical/Biological Agents and Compounds. Army Field Manual 3-9, Navy Publication P-467, and Air Force Manual 355-7. Washington, D.C.: Department of the Army/Department of the Navy/Department of the Air Force.

U.S. Army, U.S. Navy, U.S. Air Force, and U.S. Marine Corps. 1995. Treatment of Chemical Agent Casualties and Conventional Military Chemical Injuries. Army Field Manual 8-285, Navy Manual P-5041, Air Force Joint Manual 44-149, and Fleet Marine Force Manual 11-11. Washington, D.C.: Department of the Army, Department of the Navy, Department of the Air Force, and Commandant Marine Corps.

U.S. Congress. 1994. Public Law 103-160, Item 502: (51) Dec. 1701. Conduct of the Chemical and Biological Defense Program. Washington, D.C.: 103rd Congress. 1994.

U.S. Marine Corps. 1999a. Joint Operational Requirements Document (ORD) for the Joint Services Lightweight Integrated Suit Technology (JSLIST) Nuclear, Biological, and Chemical Protective Garment; Change 1. Quantico, Va.: U.S. Marine Corps Combat Development Command.

U.S. Marine Corps. 1999b. Portable Collective Protection System. Available on-line: http://www.defensedaily.com/progprof/usmc/d94a3b5995f523008525627a0053ae2b.html

Wagner, G.W., and Y.C. Yang. 1998. Baking Soda, Hydrogen Peroxide, Alcohol: The Refreshing, Universal Decon for VX, GB, and HD. Paper presented at the Scientific Conference on Chemical and Biological Defense Research, Edgewood Research, Development, and Engineering Center, Aberdeen Proving Ground, Maryland, November 20, 1998.

Walther, J.D., and J.H. Thompson. 1988. Multipurpose Chemical-Biological Decontaminant (MCBD) Trade-off Study. CRDEC-TR-88107. Aberdeen Proving Ground, Md.: Chemical Research Development and Engineering Center.

Ward, F.P. 1991. Biotechnology and Biodegradation. The Woodlands, Texas: Portfolio Publishing.

Wester, R.C., and H.I. Maibach. 1983. Cutaneous pharmacokinetics: 10 steps to percutaneous absorption. Drug Metabolism Review 14: 169–205.

Wester, R.C., and H.I. Maibach. 1999a. Dermal Decontamination and Percutaneous Absorption. Pp. 241–254 in Percutaneous Absorption, 3rd ed., R.L. Bronaugh and H.I. Maibach, eds. New York: Marcel Dekker, Inc.

Wester, R.C., and H.I. Maibach. 1999b. Interrelationships in the Dose Response of Percutaneous Absorption. Pp. 297–313 in Percutaneous Absorption, 3rd ed. R.L. Bronaugh and H.I. Maibach, eds. New York: Marcel Dekker, Inc.

Wester, R.C., and H.I. Maibach. 1999c. In vivo Methods for Percutaneous Absorption Measurements. Pp. 215–227 in Percutaneous Absorption, 3rd ed. R.L. Bronaugh and H.I. Maibach, eds. New York: Marcel Dekker, Inc.

Wigger-Alberti, W., B. Maraffio, M. Wernli, and P. Elsner. 1997. Self-application of a protective cream: pitfalls of occupational skin protection. Archives of Dermatology 133: 861–864.

Wilhelm, K.P., P. Elsner, E. Berardesca, and H.I. Maibach. 1997. Bioengineering of the Skin: Skin Surface Imaging and Analysis. Boca Raton, Fla.: CRC Press.

Williams, D., C.E. Englund, A. Sucec, and M. Overson. 1995. Cognitive effects of chemical protective clothing, exercise, and antihistamine. Military Psychology 9(4): 329–358.

Williams, N.D., and A.D. Russell. 1991. Effects of some halogen-containing compounds on *Bacillus subtilis* endospores. Journal of Applied Bacteriology 70: 427–436.

Williams, R. 1998. U.S. Army NBC Training. Presentation by R. Williams, U.S. Army Chemical School, to principal investigators and members of the Advisory Panel on Strategies to Protect the Health of Deployed U.S. Forces, Task 2.3: Physical Protection and Decontamination, Ft. McClellan, Alabama, August 11, 1998.

Wormser, U., B. Brodsky, B.S. Green, R. Arad-Yellin, and A. Nyska. 1997. Protective effect of povidone-iodine ointment against skin lesions induced by sulphur and nitrogen mustards and by non-mustard vesicants. Archives of Toxicology 71: 165–170.

Yang, Y.C. 1995. Chemical reactions for neutralising chemical warfare agents. Chemical Industry 9: 334–337.

Yang, Y.C., J.A. Baker, and J.R. Ward. 1992. Decontamination of chemical warfare agents. Chemical Reviews 92: 1729–1743.

Yang, Y.C., F.J. Berg, L.L. Szafraniec, W.T. Beaudry, C.A. Bunton, and A. Kumar. 1997. Peroxyhydrolysis of nerve agent VX and model compounds and related nucleophilic reactions. Perkin Transaction 2: 607–613.

Zhai, H., and H.I. Maibach. 1996. Effect of barrier creams: human skin *in vivo*. Contact Dermatitis 35: 92–96.

Zhai, H., and H.I. Maibach. 1998. Moisturizers in preventing irritant contact dermatitis: an overview. Contact Dermatitis 38: 241–244.

Zhai, H., P. Willard, and H.I. Maibach. 1998. Evaluating skin-protective materials against contact irritants and allergens: an *in vivo* screening human model. Contact Dermatitis 38: 155–158.

Zhai, H., D.J. Buddrus, A.A. Schulz, R.C. Wester, T. Hartway, S. Serranzana, and H.I. Maibach. 1999. In vitro percutaneous absorption of sodium lauryl sulfate (SLS) in human skin decreased by quaternium-18 bentonite gels. In Vitro and Molecular Toxicology 12: 11–16.

Zuykova, E.Y. 1959. Filtration as a method of removing microbes from the air. Gigiena Sanitariya 24(6): 72–73.

Appendices

Appendix A

Funding Levels for Fiscal Years 1996–2000 for the Joint Service Chemical/Biological Defense Program

For limited distribution to:
Government Personnel and Contractors

To obtain copies contact:
Office of the Special Assistant for Gulf War Illnesses
Four Skyline Place
5113 Leesburg Pike, Suite 901
Falls Church, VA 22041-3204
Phone: 703-578-8500

Appendix B

Textiles and Garments for Chemical and Biological Protection[1]

Frank K. Ko

INTRODUCTION

Textiles and garments are important components of the soldier system. They are the soldier's second skin, the barrier between the soldier and the surrounding environment. Although the global and national political climate has changed, and defense concepts and doctrines along with them, the basic role of clothing in protecting the soldier has remained the same.

As the battlefield environment becomes increasingly complex, we need to ask the fundamental question from time to time whether textile and garment manufacturing technology are keeping pace with current and projected demands. Do we have the fiber materials to meet specific needs? Do we have the yarn technology to convert fibers to linear fibrous assemblies? Do we have the fabric formation technology to convert fibers and yarns to planar or three dimensional (3D) fibrous assemblies? Do we have the garment assembly technology to join fabrics together to form chemical-biological (CB) protective garments? Do we have the finishing and coating materials and technology for advanced CB protective garments? Do we have the detection technology to monitor the residual life of the barrier system?

---

[1]The following material was prepared for the use of the principal investigators of this study. The opinions and conclusions herein are the author's and not necessarily those of the National Research Council.

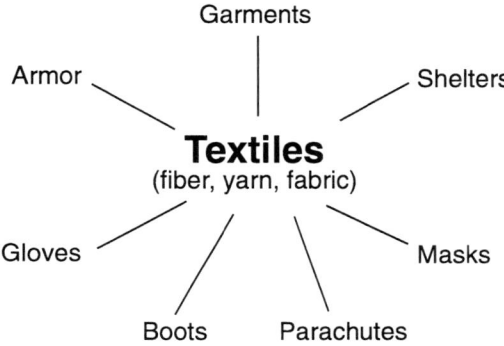

FIGURE B-1 Textiles for the protection of deployed U.S. forces. Source: U.S. Army, 1994.

Textiles are fibrous materials that include natural and synthetic fibers; linear assemblies of these fibers, such as yarn and rope; and two-dimensional (2D) and 3D assemblies of fibers in various fabric forms. These fibrous assemblies constitute the structural backbone of a broad range of military products, including garments, body armor, gloves, boots, shroud lines, masks, and shelters (see Figure B-1).

Military textiles provide battlefield, environmental, physiological, and physical protection (Table B-1). These protective functions are often required simultaneously and must not interfere with each other. For example, a barrier to protect against a chemical warfare agent must be completely impermeable, which interferes with physiological protection requirements that demand permeability to prevent heat stress.

This discussion is focused on CB protective textiles and garments. A review of the literature is followed by a description of the evolution of the requirements for CB textiles and a review of the current CB textile systems. Next, material technology (the current state of fiber, yarn, fabric, and garment technology) is assessed in terms of the nation's readiness. The performance of textile structures relevant to CB protection is expressed in terms of performance maps. On the basis of the requirements and the performance maps, development trends in CB protection are then presented. Finally, the outstanding technical issues are described.

REVIEW OF THE LITERATURE

The published literature in the public domain is limited. Information is scattered in a few chapters, monographs, and mostly in proceedings of workshops and conferences. Morris (1977), for example, summarized the

TABLE B-1 General Requirements for Protective Textiles

Battlefield Protection
    Chemical agent barrier
    Flame-resistance
    Thermal-radiation protection
    Ballistic protection
    Camouflage
    Low noise generation

Environmental Protection
    Insect proof
    Windproof
    Air-permeability insulation
    Waterproof
    Snow-shedding

Physiological Protection
    Minimum heat stress
    Windproof
    Air-permeability insulation
    Moisture-vapor permeability
    Self-sterilizing

Physical Protection
    Durability
    Low weight and bulk
    Resistance to soiling
    Self-sterilizing

Source: Morris, 1997.

requirements and classifications of protective clothing for defense purposes but only briefly discussed CB textiles.

The most relevant summary of the state of CB protective textiles was presented at an Industrial Fabric Association international conference in 1982 at which the threats of chemical warfare were described by Colonel Hidalgo of the U.S. Army Chemical School. He explained how the doctrine that led to the establishment of CB protective concepts (or fundamental principles) was formulated. The fundamental principles are: (1) contamination avoidance; (2) protection (individual and collective); and (3) decontamination (Hidalgo, 1982). These same concepts largely define the U.S. CB protection philosophy today.

Dr. Roy Roth, while working at the U.S. Army Natick Research, Development and Engineering Center (NRDEC) (now called the Soldier and Chemical Biological Command's [SBCCOM] Soldier Systems Center at

Natick) outlined the development of requirements and provided solutions and directions. Much of his discussion is still applicable today, and some concepts are just beginning to be implemented. Based on his interpretation of the Army Training and Doctrine Command's battlefield scenario, AirLand Battle 2000, Roth believed that a battlefield CB protective uniform would replace the overgarment concept of the 1970s and 1980s. He then pointed out the shortcomings of activated carbon-based protective garments (e.g., limited field life, as the activated carbon absorbs perspiration, thus depleting chemical agent sorption capabilities). Besides protection by carbon sorption, Roth introduced new concepts, such as chemical decomposition of agents and semipermeable barriers that combine sorption and decomposition.

Roth also discussed the technologies for implementing these concepts through textile materials. He focused especially on the development of multifunctional fibers, yarns, and fabrics engineering, which has led to new engineering technologies, especially melt-blown nonwoven fabrics. He also introduced the notion of a generic type of uniform for the joint service of the Army, Navy, and Air Force, which led 15 years later to the current joint service lightweight integrated suit technology (JSLIST) uniform (Roth,1982).

At the same conference, Mr. Vachon of ILC raised the issue of availability and cost of fibrous material from the contractor's point of view. He pointed out that heat stress was a problem with the microporous Teflon film, as well as the long cycle time for testing and product qualification.

To remedy the lack of research in CB protective textiles during the 1970s, several research programs were initiated by NRDEC in the 1980s. For example, to evaluate the effect of fiber architecture on the transport properties of garments, a three-year study was contracted to the Textile Research Institute, under the direction of Dr. Bernie Miller. This program resulted in a new experimental technique based on the finding that the liquid breakthrough resistance in fabric structures could be optimized by symmetric design of the fabric surface (Miller, 1986).

Considering the importance of fabric structures in CB protection, NRDEC also contracted with Drexel University, under the Textile Center of Excellence Program, to carry out a study on the feasibility of improving the performance of CB protective textiles by fabric engineering. The Drexel study revealed that the transport properties of a fabric could be engineered by modifying fabric construction, yarn materials, and yarn geometry and that a lighter and more air-permeable fabric could be designed and fabricated than the current 50/50 nylon/cotton shell fabric without sacrificing mechanical properties. Because of the lack of a quick and accurate testing method for liquid/vapor penetration, the effectiveness of the experimental fabrics for CB protection could not be tested (Ko and Geshury, 1997).

As part of the NRDEC/Drexel Textile Center of Excellence Program, an update of current CB protective concepts was presented in the 1996 Workshop on Chemical Protective Textiles jointly organized by NRDEC and Drexel University (Ko and Song, 1996). The topics covered in this workshop included barrier mechanisms for liquid and vapor agents; the characterization of barrier effectiveness based on liquid transport properties; modeling the interaction of fabric structure and physiological responses; a review of textile materials and structures for chemical protection; water and oil repellents; design of chemical protective textiles; design of chemical protective clothing; human factors in protective clothing design; and reactive systems for protection and decontamination. The workshop concluded with a projection of future protective systems and the announcement by Dr. Donald Rivin of NRDEC of the JSLIST preplanned product improvement (P3I) program.

Other sources of information on CB protective textiles are the proceedings of a series of workshops sponsored by the American Society for Testing Materials (ASTM) (McBriarty and Henry, 1992) and the ASTM special technical conference series. The ASTM articles tend to focus on test methodologies and are concerned primarily with protection in industrial environments. The Scandinavian Symposium on Protective Clothing, held every other year, covers a broad range of topics related to CB protective textiles. The role of nanotechnology in soldier protection was discussed in a recent Army workshop in Boston (Gibson and Reneker, 1998). Nanofiber structures and various reactive polymers can now be tailored for specific forms and functions.

The Army Research Office, along with other Army laboratories, has started a multidisciplinary university research initiative (MURI) involving researchers from North Carolina State University, the University of Akron, and Drexel University. Although the topics are basic in nature, the emphasis is on CB and ballistic protection.

In summary, research in CB protection textile technology was quite limited until the early 1980s when the threat of CB warfare from the Soviet bloc spurred research and development (R&D) in CB textiles and led to the development of the JSLIST garment. Considerable R&D (mostly developmental) is being conducted in the private sector, mainly on the agents and environments in industrial environments, which differ markedly from those encountered by ground soldiers. The most closely related industrial research is on protection from agricultural pesticides, which are somewhat similar to nerve agents. No significant breakthroughs in CB protective textiles are expected until new multifunctional fiber materials in a broader range of dimensional scales and structural geometries are available in an integrated design for manufacturing environments.

HISTORICAL DEVELOPMENT AND REQUIREMENTS FOR CB PROTECTIVE TEXTILES

The requirements for CB protective barriers have evolved through the years. This evolution was described in a lecture by Dr. Roy Roth (1982), which includes excellent background on the development of CB protective textiles. The following excerpt is taken from Dr. Roth's lecture:

> In the late 1960's the Army research effort had led to the development of a new biological protective clothing system. At the same time, under the Nixon administration, the government's policy to abstain from use of chemical warfare agents led to significant action. First, although the chemical biological protective clothing developed at the time was adopted by the Army in 1970, no production of the system was authorized. Such research funds as were available were committed to other higher priority projects, with virtually no funds being committed to further research in chemical protective clothing in the years thereafter.
>
> The clothing system adopted at that time was intended for ground soldiers, and more importantly it was intended to be used essentially in a defensive mode. It was a system that a soldier would use if attacked and which would permit him to move to a safe area. It was specifically not envisioned for use by ground or air combat vehicle crewmen. For most of such applications, the excessive bulk and heat stress provided by the uniform would limit the crewmen's activities.
>
> In the following seven years from 1970 to 1977, not only was relatively little research conducted in this area, but equally importantly, the battlefield scenario changed significantly. The development of a highly mechanized army employing large numbers of ground vehicles and helicopters de-emphasized the concept of the individual combat soldier covering large amounts of terrain on his own.
>
> Another change that occurred in this period was the aggressive development of chemical warfare tactics by the Soviet government. In the late 1970s it was apparent that the Soviet bloc nations were mentally, physically and emotionally equipped to use chemical biological agents in offensive modes. There was ample evidence emerging that the Soviets were organically and logistically equipped for this purpose. Down to the unit level, the Soviet army trained with and dispersed its agents, such as to make it obvious that the Soviet forces would be ready, willing, and able to use such chemical biological agents on the battlefield as if they were conventional weapons.
>
> It was equally clear that in 1977 the US was unprepared for such a situation. It is hard to imagine the nature of the obstacle confronting us in order to turn this situation around, starting with what we had. First there was a realization that chemical biological protective clothing was at best a product with substantial limitations. As noted earlier, it was

designed for defensive operations, and because of its bulk and warmth it was unsuitable for conducting extensive offensive operations, particularly in a warm environment.

We had, as noted, conducted no significant research in this area during the period 1970 to 1977. We had certainly not kept up with the times in terms of extracting what little we could from research and development in the civilian sector. On the other hand, it is an area in which little industrial research is conducted. Perhaps the nearest area of related industry activity is in the agricultural pesticides, many of which are first cousins to the nerve agents in today's military arsenal. However, little effort has been devoted to protecting against such agents in the context of an aggressive ground soldier.

To better appreciate the nature of the technical problems confronting us, we can stand back and attempt to analyze the problem in simple objective terms. Our concern is the human body, which suddenly finds itself in an alien environment comprised of an array of unwanted chemicals which are present in gaseous form, aerosol dispersed clouds, or in liquid and possibly solid form.

The eyes and the oral nasal cavities are readily accessible routes for such materials to enter the body. Some agents may be percutaneous and enter the body at any time they can reach exposed skin. The affects on the body will vary from skin inflammation to attacks on the nervous system. The end effects, depending on the agent, will run the gamut from incapacity to death. The time required to render the soldier ineffective is extremely short.

Between the soldier and a hostile environment we need a barrier, or at least a filter, that will screen out the unwanted agents. A wide variety of materials exist that provide this. However, almost all of them have one or more glaring deficiencies, which rule out their use as clothing items.

In the protective clothing area, the problem is far more complex than the typical materials research problems, which can find their solutions in sciences such as physics, chemistry, metallurgy, and so forth. When we get to clothing systems, the typical materials engineer finds himself confronted with some severe additional constraints. The materials we want must, at the very least, be able to bend and breathe in order to permit movement and avoid heat stress. Moreover, the material must be capable of being mass-produced at a reasonably low unit cost and ideally must be capable of being maintained for extended use in the field.

Among other features, it should include the ability to be camouflage printed, as well as to be laundered and decontaminated ... The material should present the strength, durability and abrasion resistance that we need for clothing in a rugged environment. Since they will be

APPENDIX B

worn in contact with the skin, there are requirements for tactile comfort and the absence of dermatological affects. Finally, the end items must be capable of withstanding extended storage under a range of temperatures and humidity without degradation.

For the ground soldier the foregoing fills many of the requirements, but for the man in combat vehicles on the ground or in the air, where a flame hazard exists, we must add the additional requirement of nonflammability.

We want to provide a barrier between the man and the environment without simultaneously creating heat stress. This would appear to present a contradiction. We want a material that is on the one hand permeable to air and body moisture vapor, and at the same time we want it to present a protective barrier to unwanted chemicals in any form.

A selective barrier is desirable, and the basic protective overgarment system we adopted in 1970 achieves this by using activated carbon in sorptive matrix to filter out the agents. The carbon is contained in a polyurethane foam matrix, which, unfortunately, carries a number of penalties, not the least of which is the heat stress it produces.

Beginning in 1978 the Natick Laboratories began rebuilding the technical base in this area, while at the same time the Defense Department began production of the CP [chemical protective] overgarments. The development of this production market stimulated interest in the research area as well. A few firms that understood the shortcomings of the current product began to turn their efforts to the problem of producing an improved overgarment material. Because of the nature of the problem and the long period of dormancy of research, we also recognized a need to have industry more completely understand both the perspective and potential that we foresaw, in hopes of stimulating still further research activities.

Within the Department of Defense, it was also recognized that the government would have to support such research, and, by 1979, several complimentary actions had been undertaken.First, Natick Laboratories and the Army Research Office conducted a seminar for industry and academic institutions to describe the problem and the potential needs. Secondly, a combined Defense Department Joint Services Technical Plan was put together with short range, intermediate, and long range objectives. In addition, a formal announcement was published in the *Commerce Business Daily* indicating the Army's initiation of a multimillion-dollar research effort, and approximately twenty-four firms indicated interest in participating in this program. Some are here represented today.

Subsequently in late 1979, eight firms responded with proposals, and research and development contracts were awarded to four major organizations. In addition, unsolicited proposals resulted in several other contracts being awarded, and the net result was a multimillion-dollar commitment to development of improved chemical protective material.

The response by industry has been heartening, and results to date are very encouraging. While many of the materials that have been produced are still being subjected to live agent testing, there is evidence that a new generation of overgarment materials may be within sight. We expect to extract from the technological base one or more materials to go into field tests in the year ahead.

The Army's Training and Doctrine Command has recently developed the scenario entitled AirLand Battle 2000. This is an attempt to look at the future in terms of the way the Army would operate in the battlefield in the year 2000 while at the same time stimulating the development of new ideas to serve the battle scene. One message that becomes clear is that we will in the future depart from today's concept of an overgarment and will be requiring a battlefield uniform that inherently possesses chemical protection. That places an unusual demand on the garment in terms of extended life in the battlefield and its ability to be maintained by conventional laundering procedures.

Today's CP [chemical protective] materials have a limited field life because a soldier's perspiration will be absorbed by the activated carbon. The greater the number of sorptive sites that are occupied by chemicals in the perspiration, the less the material will be able to absorb unwanted agents.

For this reason, the garment of the future will either have to avoid the use of activated carbon or incorporate means by which the sweat poison mechanism may be defeated or minimized. We believe it is possible to achieve the latter. There are also some signs that future generations of garments may not have to depend on activated carbon.

The overgarment existing today has this configuration: The outer shell consists of the 5-ounce nylon/cotton blended twill, the inner component, the so-called active part which contains the activated carbon impregnated into approximately a 90-mil polyurethane foam, has a liner, two-ounce nylon tricot. The bottom two layers are laminated together, and the top layer essentially floats and is put on as the garment is manufactured.

To do this, you reduce the weight in bulk, stressing again, putting this into a combat uniform configuration as opposed to a defensive mode, increase shelf life, adding fire retardancy as best we can, particularly for tank and air crewmen, and making it launderable. It should be launderable not only in combination with being decontaminated, should there be a threat, but since it hopefully will be the combat uniform it should be launderable during the time that it is being worn when there is no threat . . .

APPENDIX B

Durability, camouflage, you tend to look at this whole thing, remember Alec Guinness and the man in the white suit. Well, we can't even do that, we have to have camouflaging to go along with it. Water repellency, as I mentioned, perspiration resistance and petroleum products, nontoxic as far as materials go and compatibility with other items, ... whether they be a backpack or a detection kit and so forth. It must all be compatible with those systems, too.

There are many different material systems being investigated to attempt to achieve these objectives. ... Some of them are based on active carbon power, some of them are based on active fiber yarn, some of them are based on what I call barrier film.

Perhaps a simpler way of demonstrating the scope of the program is to sort out the various efforts in terms of mechanisms or approaches involved. These are the three broad categories, which comprise the technical approaches that exist right now. Approach one is based on sorptivity, using activated carbon in various forms. Approach two is based on trying to develop and put into a uniform some way of actually destroying the chemical threat by decomposition. Number three, is based on either a combination of the above or individually a barrier of some sort ... in the first category, based on carbon powder. Instead of the polyurethane foams other possible foams might have advantages, being more permeable, being substantive to the carbon, etc., so that the activity of the carbon may remain higher.

Technology allows us to make hollow fibers into which we could put activated carbon powder. Technology permits us to make fibers *in situ* along with carbon powder. Essentially you would be laying down a web of material. Technology permits putting in carbon powder along with melt-blown materials such as polypropylene. I draw particular attention to ... what I call the nonwoven area, which I think would have some very interesting possibilities.

From the carbon fiber standpoint, this is also being pursued. In general it is noted or to emphasize the expense increases as we go from powder to fiber and within fiber from staple down to fabric. [There] are different forms of carbon fiber, using staple. It can be done by conventional techniques, putting down either wet laid or dry laid nonwovens. We can flock carbon fiber onto various substrates. We can make engineered fabrics out of carbon yarn either with other materials to strengthen it or in other configurations. We can start with fabrics, which are one hundred percent activated carbon and use it somehow. It is fairly weak and brittle to begin with, so it would have to be protected.

Presently carbon fiber is not available in any reasonable quantity domestically. It is only available overseas (Japan or England), and that is a deficiency. If this approach is successful, we would have to have a domestic source.

The second broad category, protection by chemical decomposition, is not new in concept but is new in terms of materials and technology we are applying to the problem. These approaches may hold an answer to some of the longer range needs. It has been known in the literature that there are materials that can hydrolyze the threats. It has been shown that certain ion-exchange resins will do this. It is a question of how we incorporate them into a fabric, and are they active enough to really decompose the threat during a dynamic situation.

There has been recent publicity about some enzymes that have been isolated primarily from squid, which are known to hydrolyze certain live agents. We have the same question. Is it possible to immobilize these somehow and attach them to fabrics, and if so, will it have all of the other properties that are needed, that were listed earlier?

You begin to think, well, are these possible to launder, to decontaminate, etc. Finally, there are efforts directed to the third approach. It reflects an attempt to combine some of the foregoing approaches by developing an engineered material system. Given the present and expected future threat, representing an array of different agents, such a system would have growth potential, which is necessary given the rapidly changing technological world in which we live.

Ideally, of course, it would be nice to have a semipermeable barrier that will keep out the agents and will breathe, will allow moisture vapor to go through and from a waterproofing standpoint will keep out liquid water. Ideally, as I say, it would be better to have that without the need for an absorptive material.

I think most of the approaches and techniques, which I talked about, can tend to identify here. It is best to go around them again to repeat them, starting with carbon, putting carbon powder again into a textile material, whether it be embedded in the fiber or in a hollow fiber, trying to use carbon fibers in one form or another. Your approach of using reactive materials, whether they be, for example, ion-exchange resins, is more of the idealized situation that I just mentioned as a possibility.

On the next one, the barrier film actually exists right now. That's the composition of the butyl rubber overboot and is the system, which the Soviets have gone toward. Unfortunately, it maximizes heat stress and is completely impermeable, which is not a desirable situation for a combat uniform.

Another possibility is using activated fibers again, laminated structures and the possibility of using nonwovens in one form or another.

The impetus given to this program and the results to date will lead to continued funding of research and development efforts in chemical protection material. From a production standpoint, there is no question that a significantly improved chemical production uniform would produce in itself a sizeable market.

In the period 1977 to 1981, we procured approximately six million chemical protected overgarments, which cost about $188 million. In time, these garments will have to be replaced, and thus a sizeable market looms ahead. If we had a CP uniform today that could be used as an everyday battle uniform with the requisite field life and ease of maintainability, this would certainly stimulate this process and lead to additional procurement.

. . . [T]he Army, Navy, and Air Force have some specific needs for chemical protection, but it is distinctly possible that a system offering minimum heat stress, which would include flame resistance, would be universally adopted by all services. Also, the possibility of the allied forces incorporating and improved system exists, too.

In previous comments I have addressed the chemical protective uniform as opposed to the other components such as footwear, headwear, and mask. For your information the mask and so forth are the responsibilities of the Chemical Systems Laboratories where the remaining part of the uniform are their responsibility, including the gloves and the overboots of the Natick Laboratories.

The footwear and handwear represent another opportunity in that today's products are impermeable butyl rubber, which in the case of handwear, represents significant problems of loss of tactical sense. There is no question that we want to develop handwear that provides the minimum encumbrances and maximum tactical sense possible. Although much of our effort to date has concentrated on protective clothing, a separate initiative has been undertaken to develop highly tactile gloves. In this area, in which materials research people who have familiarity with the elastomer technology will probably be best equipped to handle this task.

Our current butyl rubber items, I might add, also have a flammability problem, which we wish to avoid in the future. This is another material characteristic that would be desired not only for handwear but also for footwear and hood materials, which cover the head area.

The technical requirements for CB protective textiles described by Dr. Roth, which are summarized in Table B-2, can be further divided into five key properties: weight, bulk, durability (wear time-protection time), comfort, and heat stress. The specific requirements of these properties were quantified in a recent presentation by Mr. Phil Brandler of SBCCOM's Soldier Systems Center (1998), who projected the need for a substantial reduction in weight with the ultimate goals of indefinite wear and self-

TABLE B-2 Requirements for Chemical
Protective Textiles

Reduced heat stress
Reduced weight-to-bulk ratio
Combat uniform configuration
Longer service life
Longer shelf life
Fire resistance
Laundering capability
Decontamination capability
Reusability
Durability
Camouflage capability
Water repellency
Perspiration resistance
Resistance to petroleum products
Nontoxic materials
Compatible with other items

Source: Roth, 1982.

decontamination. Table B-3 summarizes the evolution of the durability and weight requirements of CB protective garments.

CURRENT BARRIER SYSTEMS

The current U.S. Army chemical protective battle-dress overgarment (BDO) is a composite structure consisting of an outer shell, an inner activated-carbon layer, and a liner (Figure B-2). The outer shell consists of 7oz/yd^2 nylon/cotton blend in a twist weave construction; the liner is a lighter (2 oz/yd^2) nylon tricot warp knit structure.

Reducing weight and bulk, improving durability, and reducing heat stress will require assessing the entire inventory of textile materials, including fibers, yarn, and fabric structures. Weight can be reduced by using fibers of lower density and yarn and fabric structures with low packing density. Bulk can be reduced by using smaller diameter fibers with higher packing density. The durability of the garment can be improved with stronger and tougher fibers and improved fabric construction (e.g., optimal interlacing density). To improve fabric comfort or reduce heat stress, the permeability and thermal conductivity of the fiber and structure can be increased. Table B-4 summarizes the general improvements in material properties required to achieve textile design goals.

The individual can be protected against chemical agents by an impermeable barrier or by a selectively semipermeable barrier. Materials that

TABLE B-3 Evolution of Performance Requirements for Protective Textiles

1960s	XXCC3 underwear	7 days wear 6 hours protection
1970s	Chemical protective overgarment	14 days wear 6 hours protection
1980s	Overgarment84/BDO	22 days wear 24 hours protection
1990s	JSLIST	45 days wear 24 hours protection
2000s	JSLIST P31	60 days wear 24 hours protection
AAN	ICS	indefinite wear self-decontaminating

Source: Brandler, 1998.

create a physically impermeable barrier to chemical agents are also impermeable to moisture. Impermeable barrier materials, such as rubber and coated fabrics, do not allow enough moisture-vapor permeability to be useful. The effective period of use of impermeable barrier materials is very limited because of heat stress. The impermeable barrier approach was used for protective clothing until the mid-1970s. Currently, it is used only for gloves, boots, and other special applications intended for short-time use, such as the suit, contamination avoidance, liquid protection (SCALP), the toxicological agent protective (TAP) outfit, and the self-contained toxic environment protective outfit (STEPO).

The second approach can be either (1) a semipermeable fabric and a sorptive layer that can filter out/decompose chemical agents or

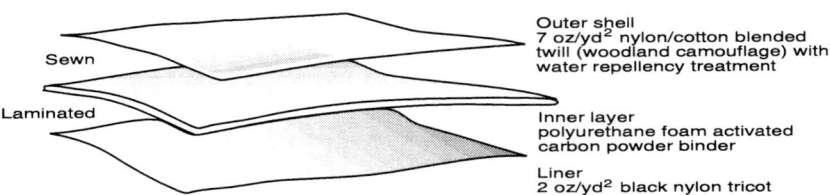

FIGURE B-2 Components of a typical barrier system.

TABLE B-4 Summary of Required Improvements in Material Properties

Needs	Properties
Decreased weight	Decreased fiber specific gravity Decreased packing density
Decreased bulk	Decreased fiber diameter Increased packing density
Increased durability	Increased strength, toughness
Increased comfort	Increased permeability
Decreased heat stress	Increased thermal conductivity

Source: Ko, 1999.

(2) selectively permeable/membrane materials. The sorptive layer involves using activated carbon (powder or fibers) to adsorb agent. Carbon powder can be in the form of foam, coated fibers, hollow fibers, or meltblown fibers. Activated carbon fibers can be used as nonwoven, flocked fabrics or laminated structures. Chemical decomposition of agents can be achieved through the use of reactive resins or reactive enzymes. The selective permeable/membrane concept is the focus of current R&D by SBCCOM's Soldier Systems Center (Figure B-3).

The current standard U.S. Army chemical protective BDO has the following configuration: the outer shell consists of 7 oz/yd^2 nylon/cotton blended twill (woodland camouflage) or around 6 oz/yd^2 triblend (cotton/nylon/Kevlar) twill (desert camouflage) with water repellent treatment. The inner layer contains the activated carbon impregnated into approximately a 90-mil polyurethane foam laminated to a 2 oz/yd^2 nylon tricot liner. The inner layer components are laminated together. The top layer essentially floats and is put on as the garment is manufactured.

The aircrew uniform integrated battlefield (AUIB) combines CB protection with flame resistance with an outer shell made of 95 percent Nomex and 5 percent Kevlar. The inner layer is similar to the inner layer of the BDO. Clothing used by the Marine Corps, the Saratoga, is a CB protective suit with carbon sphere. An alternative to the BDO, the Saratoga can be worn over normal duty uniforms.

The JSLIST Program was completed recently and is currently progressing to the JLIST P3I. The purpose of these programs was to develop the next generation of chemical protective clothing ensembles by consolidating ongoing efforts: (1) to provide the best suit(s) possible for each service (Air Force, Army, Marines, and Navy); (2) to minimize the types

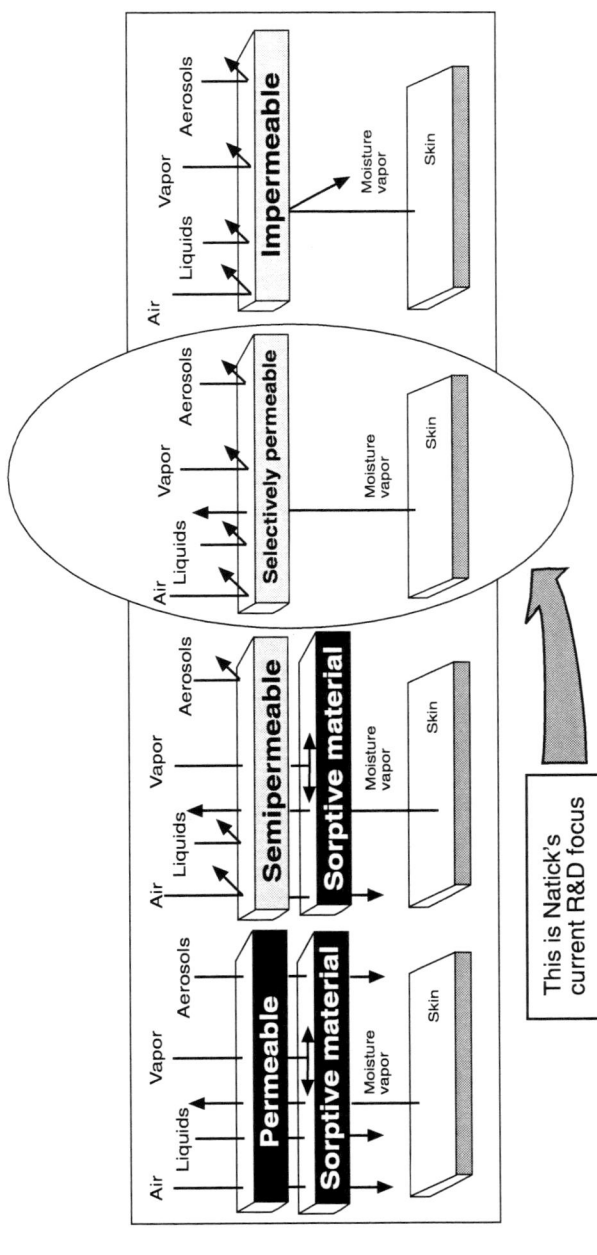

FIGURE B-3 Selectively semipermeable barrier construction. Source: Wilusz, 1998.

of suits in service; (3) to maximize economies of scale; and (4) to conserve service resources.

The JSLIST overgarment is a universal, lightweight, two-piece, front-opening garment that can be worn as an overgarment or as a primary uniform over personal underwear. It has an integral hood, bellows-type sockets, high-waist trousers, adjustable suspenders, adjustable waistband, and waist-length jacket. This overgarment is more comfortable and more readily accepted and is compatible with other equipment.

The JSLIST overgarment provides optimum protection against vapor and aerosol agents, as well as liquid resistance. It is fully compatible with the extreme cold weather clothing system; the improved chemical and biological protective gloves; the multipurpose overboot; the M17, M40, M43, and MCU2P series protective masks; protective masks currently under development, including the XM45; clothing and individual equipment; and developmental individual soldier and marine systems, including the next-generation family of body armor, Generation 11 systems, and Land Warrior systems. The key features of the JSLIST overgarment include: CB agent protection; reduced heat stress; launderability; enhanced durability; improved capability; and improved comfort (Barrett, 1998).

The system is now available in several different configurations through the United States licensee, Tex-Shield, Inc. The Saratoga system, which uses encapsulated active-carbon spheres, has demonstrated lower heat stress, higher air permeability, repeated laundering, resistance to perspiration and petroleum products, nonflammability, good strength, and less bulk (Gander, 1997).

An integral part of the development of chemical protective clothing is the development of testing and evaluation methods for assessing the performance of chemical protective clothing under simulated conditions that are as realistic as possible. Tests for evaluating the effectiveness of barrier systems vary from simple small-scale swatch tests to full-scale field tests (NRC, 1997).

TEXTILE MATERIALS

Fibers

Textile fibers are slender, flexible, and have a length-to-diameter ratio of 1,000:1. Beside flexibility, the unique characteristic of textile fibers is a combination of strength, light weight, and toughness. The strength of fibers ranges from 1 gram per denier (g/den) to 40 g/den for super high-strength fibers. Elongation ranges from 1 percent to several hundred percent for elastomers.

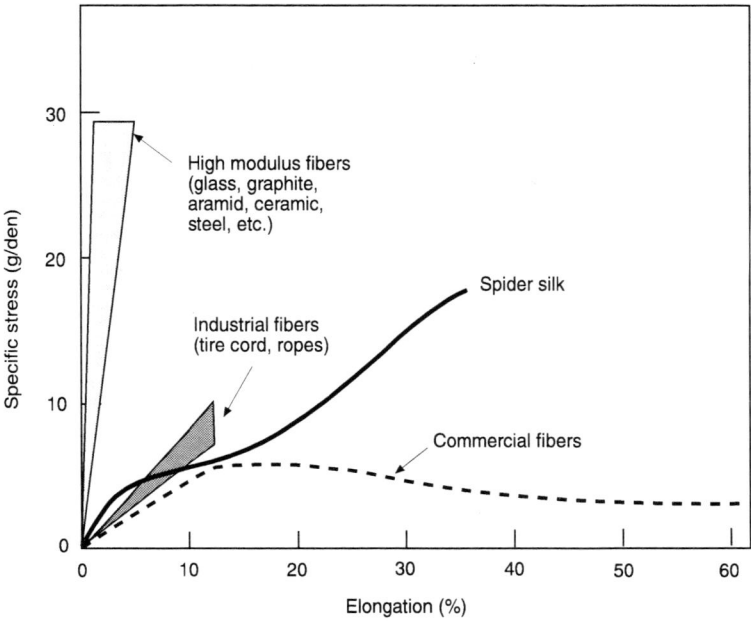

FIGURE B-4 Stress-strain curves of natural and man-made fibers. Source: Ko, 1999.

The stress-strain properties of fibers depend on their chemical composition and internal structures. The stress-strain curves of natural and man-made fibers show the wide range of material properties available (Figure B-4). The fiber with the best combination of strength and toughness is spider silk. Therefore, spider silk has been selected as the model for the fiber of the future for soldier protection. Textile fibers are classified according to their geometry, chemical composition, or thermomechanical properties (Table B-5).

Natural fibers include wool, silk, and asbestos; man-made fibers include rayon, aramid, and graphite. Fibers may be categorized as organic or inorganic on the basis of their hydrocarbon composition. Most general-purpose textile fibers are organic; most high-performance fibers are inorganic. Thermoplastic and thermoset fibers are defined based on their response to temperature. Thermoplastic fibers, such as polyester or nylon, can be formed and reshaped under temperatures higher than their solidification, or setting, temperatures. Thermoset, such as rayon and epoxy-based fibers, once set, cannot be changed. Fibers are classified as regular,

TABLE B-5 Physical and Mechanical Properties of Textile Fibers

Fiber	Density (g/cc)	Strength (g/denier)	Modulus (g/denier)	Elongation (%)	Melting Temp (°C)	Moisture Regain (%)
Polypropylene	0.90	3.5	20.0	70.0	160	0.01
Polyethylene (Spectra)	0.97	30.0	1400.0	3.6	143	0
Nylon	1.14	3.5	17.0	16.0	248	4.0
Modacrylic	1.18	1.7	3.8	45.0	(198)	2.5
Wool	1.31	1.0	4.5	25.0	(298)	16.0
Polyester	1.38	2.8	12.0	12.0	250	0.4
Aramid (Kevlar 29)	1.44	23.0	500.0	4.0	(482)	4.3
Rayon	1.52	2.3	60.0	10.0	(176)	
Cotton	1.54	3.0	60.0	3.0	(149)	8.5
Carbon	1.78	24.0	1,500.0	1.6	N/A	N/A
Teflon	2.2	0.9	1.0	19.0	326	0
E-glass	2.54	15.3	320.0	4.8	1,120	0

Source: Ko and Song, 1996.

medium, high, or super-high tenacity according to their responses to tensile loading.

General Properties of Fibers

The structure and properties of textile fibers have been the subject of several books over the past 40 years. The first treatment of fibers as an engineering material was presented by Dewitt Smith in his ATSM Edgar Marburg Lecture (DeWitt Smith, 1944). As the development of synthetic fibers continued, Harris and his associates at the Harris Research Laboratories compiled an impressive collection of physical and mechanical properties of textile fibers (Harris, 1954). Moncrieff (1963) gave a comprehensive description of the function of commercial fibers emphasizing the technological, experimental, and economic aspects of fiber development. Herman Mark et al. (1967) edited a three-volume treatise on man-made fibers. Expanding on the 1962 edition of their book, Morton and Hearle (1975) published a textbook on the physical properties of textile fibers representing the most up-to-date discussion of the structure, properties, and characterization of fibers.

Physical Properties of Conventional Textile Fibers

Thermal Properties

Thermal properties include melting temperature, softening temperature, and decomposition temperature. These properties indicate how well a fiber can withstand the temperature for use. As a general textile, it should have a melting point higher than 200°C. Melting temperatures range from 140°C for polypropylene to 800°C for glass to 3,600°C for graphite.

Moisture Absorption

The water absorption characteristics of fibers are usually expressed in terms of moisture regain. Because the moisture content of fibers affects the weight, moisture regain is an important consideration for fiber users. Moisture in a fiber also affects its mechanical properties, comfort, and processability. Hydrophilic fibers absorb water readily; hydrophobic fibers absorb little or no water. Moisture regain is computed by the following equation:

$$mosture\ regain = \frac{conditioned\ weight - dry\ weight}{dry\ weight} \times 100\%$$

The amount of moisture a fiber absorbs depends on the presence of polar groups and the availability of these groups within the amorphous regions of the fiber. The principal water-binding groups in fibers include the hydroxyl, carboxyl, carbonyl, and amino groups. Natural cellulosic fibers are usually more hydrophilic than synthetic fibers. Moisture regain ranges from 0 percent for hydrophobic fibers like glass and polypropylene to 16 percent for hydrophilic fibers like wool.

Electrical Properties

The electrical resistance of a fiber depends on the humidity of the atmosphere and the nature of the polymer. Fibers of high electrical resistance are prone to "static" problems. The generation of static electricity causes difficulty in textile processes, such as yarn spinning, weaving, and knitting. Static also causes garments to cling and makes soil removal difficult in laundering and dry cleaning. Cellulosic fibers have low electrical resistance; synthetic fibers have high electrical resistance. Electrical resistance ranges from 6.8 Ω kg/m^2 (ohm kilogram per square meter) for cotton to 14 Ω kg/m^2 for polyester and acrylic.

Fiber Geometry

The surface geometry of fibers can be characterized by roughness, cross-sectional shape, and crimp. Surface geometry affects the frictional characteristics, luster, bulkiness, and flexibility of a fiber. Fiber geometry affects the appearance of textile structures, the processability of fibers, and the handling and mechanical properties of fabrics. Most natural fibers have rough surfaces and irregular cross-sectional shape and crimp. The cross-sectional shape of synthetic fibers ranges from round to irregular; the cross-sectional shape of some fibers can be modified to change their working characteristics. Delustrants are usually added to increase the surface roughness of synthetic fibers.

The fineness of the fiber has the most influence on the performance of CB protective textiles. Fiber diameters range from 20–26 microns for wool to 0.001 microns for electrospun fibers (Fukuhara, 1993). Microfibers can be produced by drawing, islands-in-the-sea (when a particular fiber contains individual smaller fibers of one polymer spun inside a matrix, or sea, of another fiber), radial sheath separation, or multilayer separate processes. Toray (a leading Japanese producer) has reported that fiber diameters as fine as 0.1 micron (0.0001 denier) have been successfully produced in the laboratory (Fukuhara, 1993). Recently, du Pont also introduced a textile microfiber. Most microfibers are for garment applications.

A microdenier carbon fiber (Pyrograf) produced by GM by the vapor-grown process has a diameter of 0.2 microns, which increases the available fiber surface. The finest fibers that have been demonstrated, however, are produced by the electrospinning process. In this process, a polymer solution is exposed to an electrical field that elongates the polymer jet to form fibers ranging from 50 to 150 nm in diameter (Reneker and Chun, 1996). A wide range of polymers have been demonstrated successfully in Dr. Reneker's laboratory at Akron, at the Fibrous Materials Research Center at Drexel University, and at several government laboratories (Gibson et al., 1999; Ko et al., 1998).

Different functionalities can be introduced to the fibers (i.e., activated carbon imbedded fibers, hollow fibers filled with activated carbon, activated carbon overbraided with cotton, activated carbon-coated yarns, and reactive fibers) by texturing, polymer modification, special sizing, denier mixing, sludge mixing, coating, wrapping, and chemical treatment. The combination of nanofiber with microfiber or regular multifilament fibers is a new program being initiated in the Drexel-Akron part of the Army MURI program. A wide range of bulkiness and mechanical properties can be engineered into a fiber.

Yarns

A yarn is a continuous strand of textile fiber or filaments in a form suitable for knitting, weaving, or intertwining to form textile fabrics. The formation system depends on the nature of the fiber (natural or manmade; long or short; fine or coarse) and the end-use requirements. The fiber material properties and the geometry (e.g., twist, denier, etc.) determine the performance properties of a yarn and consequently, dictate the processing methods and applications for which a yarn is suited. For the implemented technology of yarns, readers are encouraged to consult Goswami et al. (1971) and Kaswell (1965). Yarns can be classified according to form, by formation system, or by physical properties and performance characteristics.

State of the Art of Fibers and Yarns

The fiber and textile industries have made a good deal of progress in the production of fibers and yarns, especially in Japan and Europe whose textile machine industries dominate the world market (Berkowitch, 1996). The following excerpts from Berkowitch's review describe advances in Japanese industry.

> Driven by the desire to lower cost and increase uniformity of synthetic fibers, eight producers participated in a six-year MITI funded project that ended in 1988. The project was designed, among other things, to raise polyester spinning speed beyond 6,000 m per minute. ...these advances resulted in an abundant patent literature and lowered the rate of yarn breaks by a factor of 100 (down to 1 or 2 per 10^8 m), making it possible to operate continuously at 6,000 m per minute for 12 days. They allow easy spinning in the range of 6,000 to 8,000 m per minute. The participating producers incidentally designed and built most of the equipment required for the improvements, including winders.
>
> As a result of the project, producers now can use either a pressurized compartment or a compressed air circulation arrangement to sequentially draw and false-twist texture polyesters at wind-up speeds exceeding 2,000 m per minute.
>
> Still another outcome of the MITI project was the clustered spinning of several (three to ten) yarn ends into a single spinning block. Circular air flow delivered perpendicularly to the spinning direction quenches the bundles of filaments, which may range from 0.8 to 8 deniers. Winding takes place at speeds anywhere from 3,000 to 8,000 m per minute.
>
> Today, automation of the spinning process has reduced the amount of labor to the point where major producers have essentially unmanned polyester and nylon production lines.

Berkowitch goes on to predict that Korean industry is following suit. Another innovation in Japanese industry is flexibility in manufacturing systems.

> The growth of the specialty fiber business prompted producers to increase the flexibility of their facilities. Streams of homopolyester coming from continuous polymerizers are now split into substreams, each modified by injecting additives, such as pigments, lubricants, and hydrophilic and antimicrobial agents, and each homogenized with in-line static mixers to produce parallel yarn ends of different compositions in small volumes.
>
> The review of conjugate-spun products outlined the spinning of filaments that contain two or more distinct polymer phases. Once in fabrics, the yarns are subjected to one of four finishing procedures, depending on their composition and targeted end use. The first, heat setting after bleaching and dyeing, does not alter the macrostructure of the filaments. It only stabilizes the dimensions of the fabric, which has the attributes brought about by the additive used in one of the two polymer phases. The second, heat relaxation, lets the individual filaments self-crimp according to the asymmetry and difference of shrinkage

potential that exists between the two phases. It also confers stretch. The third, generally an alkaline treatment, dissolves one of the phases freeing the other. The fourth, mechanical fibrillation, subdivides the filaments longitudinally, capitalizing on a designed low-phase adhesion. The last two produce sub-denier filaments, leading to novel aesthetics and functionalities.

The cross-section geometry of a conjugate-spun filament mirrors the shape, size, and relative position of the small orifices from which the various polymer streams emerge immediately prior to their coalescence. The range of numerical values these variables can take, not to mention the diversity of polymer compositions, opens the door to a practically unlimited number of combinations and thus products.

Berkowitch also described fluid-based processing techniques.

Fluid-processing techniques (air, steam, or water) are broadly found in textiles worldwide as substitutes for mechanical devices offering high productivity and labor savings. The turbulence created by impinging products with fluids alters their structures in a desirable way. This action takes place inside jets, as with air in consolidating filament bundles by interlacing; bulking yarns by crimping and looping; or forming staple yarns by entangling and wrapping. In another series of embodiments, pressurized water exiting from jets generates subdenier filaments by fibrillation), forms nonwoven fabrics by fiber lacing, and propels fill yarns across warps on waterjet looms.

One Japanese textile equipment manufacturer pioneered a staple yarn formation process that uses two air-driven torque jets operating in series, but with the directions of their vortices opposite to each other. Fabrics made from such yarns tend to have a harsh hand and, for that reason, have been frowned on by the domestic market. However, other countries (the United States in particular), driven by the attractive economics, have commercialized the process and continue to seek improvements by fine-tuning feed fiber specifications. With growing cost sensitization, the Japanese textile industry may soon start adding to the 2,500 machines already in use abroad.

Fabrics

Although there are numerous possibilities for fabric geometries, most fabrics are formed by the three basic systems: (1) weaving (interlacing two or more systems of yarns); (2) knitting (interlooping one or more yarns); (3) chemical or mechanical bonding of fibers for nonwoven fabrics. As a rule of thumb, knitting is approximately 10 times faster than weaving, and nonwoven fabrics can be made about 100 times faster than woven fabrics.

Fabric Performance Characteristics

Fabric performance characteristics are based on the interaction between fiber (material properties), yarn, fabric geometry, and finishing treatment. Obvious characteristics of fabrics for textile applications are: (1) comfort; (2) aesthetic value; (3) functionality and durability; and (4) ease of care.

Garments

The garments and protective textile structures for the soldier are produced by direct fiber-to-fabric or yarn-to-fiber processes. Yarn-to-fabric structures include woven and knitted fabrics. Fiber-to-fabric structures are known as nonwoven structures. A wide variety of fiber architectures can be generated from the three basic fabric processes (weaving, knitting, and bonding), resulting in a wide range of interlacing (bonding) density, fiber orientation/distribution, and formability/conformability. For example, woven fabrics include biaxial, triaxial, and multiaxial interlacing of yarns; and interlacing density varies from high density in the plain weave construction to low density in the satin weave construction. Knitted structures (interlooped structures) are characterized by high porosity and conformability. Knits are classified into warp knits (yarns are introduced across the machine) and weft knits (yarns are introduced along the machine). The openness of knitted structures can be reduced and the stability of the structure enhanced by the insertion of directional yarn. Inserted yarns can be organized from unidirectional, orthogonal, and bidirectional to multidirectional.

Nonwoven structures are primarily formed by direct conversion of fiber-to-fabric by mechanical or chemical bonding. These fiber-based structures are characterized by high areal coverage to areal density ratio. Nonwoven fabrics are extremely versatile because they can combine fiber-based and yarn-based structures. Mechanically bonded nonwoven fabrics can be produced by needling or fluid-jet entanglement. These structures tend to be bulky but quite conformable. Chemically bonded nonwoven fabrics are less bulky but tend to be paper-like and nonconformable. Because of the simplicity of processing and high productivity of nonwoven fabrics, industry has a strong incentive to use nonwoven structures for primary garment fabrics. However, their paper-like consistency has been a major obstacle to the popular acceptance of nonwoven structures.

The current JSLIST garment is a combination of all three textile structures. Woven structures are used in the shell; the liner is warp knitted; and the structure that carries the activated carbon absorbents is a nonwoven fabric (or foam).

Automated Garment Manufacturing

The automation of garment manufacturing in the United States is well behind that of Japan. Complete automation of the tailored apparel manufacturing system was developed in Japan under a nine year Ministry of International Trade and Industry funded contract begun in 1982. According to Berkowitch (1996):

> A consortium of 28 enterprises from all segments of the industry cooperated in the project. The seed for the initiative lay in the uncertain future faced by a labor-intensive, low-tech industry in a high-wage economy and in the potential for a domestic production capability that had low labor requirements and was flexible, just in time, and quality oriented. The undertaking was ambitious—it called for having a bolt of cloth at one end and tailored garments ready for shipment at the other, without the intervention of human hands in between. It anticipated that manufacturing time would be cut in half. Technically, the challenge was to apply robotics to the manufacture of sophisticated sewn articles using diverse flexible materials. By the time the project concluded in 1990, essentially all process elements had been demonstrated in the production of tailored women's jackets of woven and knit cloths, patterned and dyed in solid colors.

In the future, individual modules of the production line optimized for making specific garments or garment parts are likely to find their way into the domestic industry in Japan.

Fabric Performance Maps

The properties of textile structures can be characterized in terms of geometric and performance properties critical to CB protection. The performance maps outline the region of performance of various fabrics. To facilitate comparisons on the same basis, the fabric performance maps for yarn-to-fabric and fiber-to-fabric structures are discussed separately. Because of the broad range of possibilities, the performance maps are qualitative, rather than quantitative.

Critical Properties

The properties included in the performance maps reflect the basic requirements of CB protective textiles: (1) reduction in weight; (2) reduction in bulk; (3) reduction of heat stress (increased comfort); and (4) increased durability. These requirements can be translated into four geometric parameters and four performance parameters. The geometric parameters include:

- *Porosity* (the amount of open space in a unit volume of fabric). As fiber diameter and yarn diameter increase, the structure tends to become more porous. The porosity of a fabric is inversely proportional to the areal coverage or cover factor of a fabric. A porous fabric tends to be lighter and more permeable than a nonporous fabric.
- *Surface Texture.* The surface geometry of a fabric is characterized by the smoothness of the surface, which in turn is governed by fiber and yarn diameter.
- *Voluminosity* (a reflection of the bulkiness of a fabric for a given areal density [mass per unit area]). A fabric tends to be more voluminous if the fiber/yarn diameter is larger and the freedom of fiber mobility in the geometric repeating unit is high. Voluminosity is directly related to fiber thickness.
- *Thickness of the fabric.* Like voluminosity, thickness is related to fiber and yarn diameter. The larger the fiber and yarn diameter, the thicker and bulkier the fabric.

The performance parameters include:

- *Permeability* (the ease of air or liquid flow through a fabric). The permeability of a fabric increases when the porosity increases.
- *Compressibility* (the ability of a fabric to resist transverse [through the thickness] compression). A voluminous fabric tends to be more compressible than a nonvoluminous fabric. Compressibility decreases with the stiffness of the fiber and yarn, which is significantly influenced by fiber diameter. As fiber diameter increases, the bending stiffness and longitudinal compressive stiffness of the fiber increases geometrically.
- *Extensibility* (the ability of a fabric to stretch and conform). Fabric extensibility is affected by fabric geometry and inherent fiber bending elongation.
- *Toughness* (the durability of the fabric). A high-strength fabric with high elongation at break usually has high toughness.

Yarn-to-Fabric Structures

Interlooped structures, such as weft knits, tend to be more porous, more voluminous, and bulkier and thicker than other yarn-to-fabric structures. Interlaced structures, such as woven fabrics, tend to be less porous, less bulky, and thinner. The performance of all yarn-to-fabric structures is largely determined by the linearity and interlacing density of the yarns. For example, weft knits have high extensibility, are extremely comfortable, and are very compressible. Because of the openness of the loop geometry, weft knits are highly permeable. Because of the high linearity of the multiaxial (noncrimped) warp knit structure, these fabrics have limited extensibility and low toughness. The permeabilities of woven and multiaxial warp knit fabrics are lower than those of weft knit fabrics. Figures B-5 and B-6 show the qualitative performance maps for the geometric and performance properties of the yarn and fabric.

Fiber-to-Fabric Structures

Fiber-to-fabric structures are generally known as nonwoven fabrics. The simplicity of the manufacturing processes by which fibers are converted directly to fabrics (thus bypassing the yarn-formation stage) has great appeal to the industry (especially the apparel industry) because of high productivity and cost savings. But nonwoven fabrics do not have good drapability/conformability characteristics. Of the two major classes of nonwoven fabrics (chemically bonded and mechanically bonded), mechanically bonded systems (e.g., needle felts and spunlaced systems) tend to be more voluminous, bulkier, thicker, and more porous. Chemically bonded nonwoven fabrics tend to be more paper-like, thin, nonbulky, and less porous. As a result, mechanically bonded nonwoven fabrics are more permeable, more extensible, and more compressible.

The performance map shows only a partial view of the toughness of nonwoven fabrics. A spun-bonded system, because of the high strength of the continuous filaments and the strength of the bonds, has a high level of shear resistance, tear resistance, and toughness. The needle felt fiber (e.g., Kevlar), can also be quite tough, even capable of arresting fragments from a ballistic projectile.

A summary of the performance map of fiber-to-fabric structures is shown in Figures B-7 and B-8. The effect of fiber orientation (fiber architecture) on permeability is illustrated in Figure B-9. Nonwoven fabric, because of its torturous fiber architecture, is significantly less permeable than woven fabric under the same fiber volume fraction. In nonwoven fabrics, fiber dimension engineering can further modify coverage or porosity. Finer fibers provide significantly higher fabric coverage (Ko and Pastore, 1985). Based on the general performance map, experimental evidence, and simulated results, we can conclude that fiber architecture and fiber diameter are very important in controlling the geometric and performance characteristics important for CB protective textiles.

FUTURE DIRECTIONS

The requirements for the next generation of CB protective garments

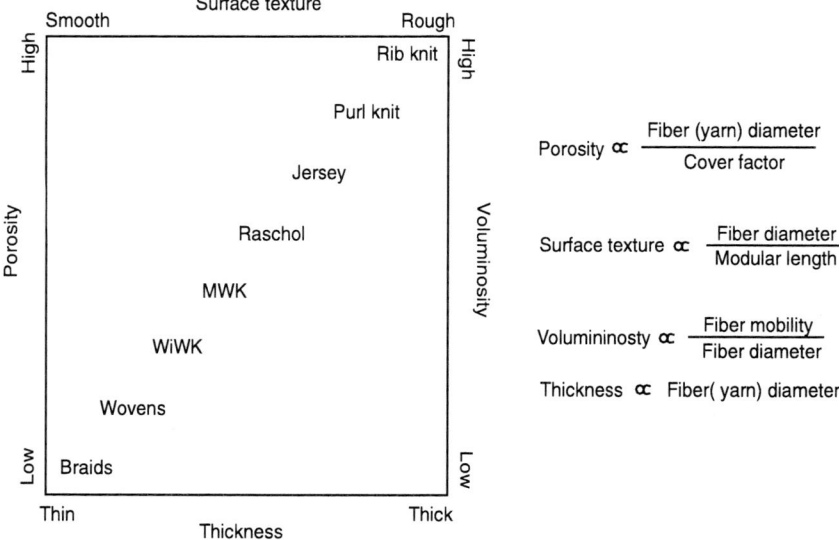

FIGURE B-5 Geometric properties of knit and woven fibers. Source: Ko and Song, 1996.

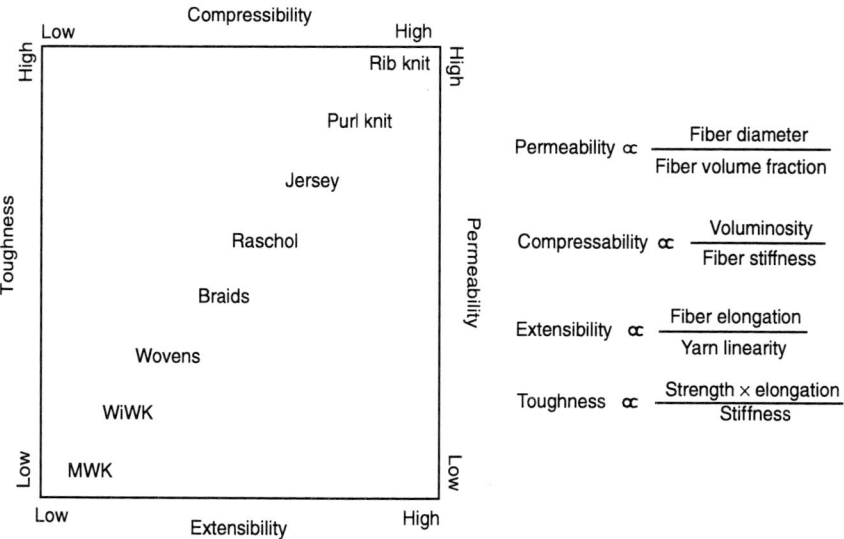

FIGURE B-6 Performance properties of knit and woven fibers. Source: Ko and Song, 1996.

APPENDIX B   211

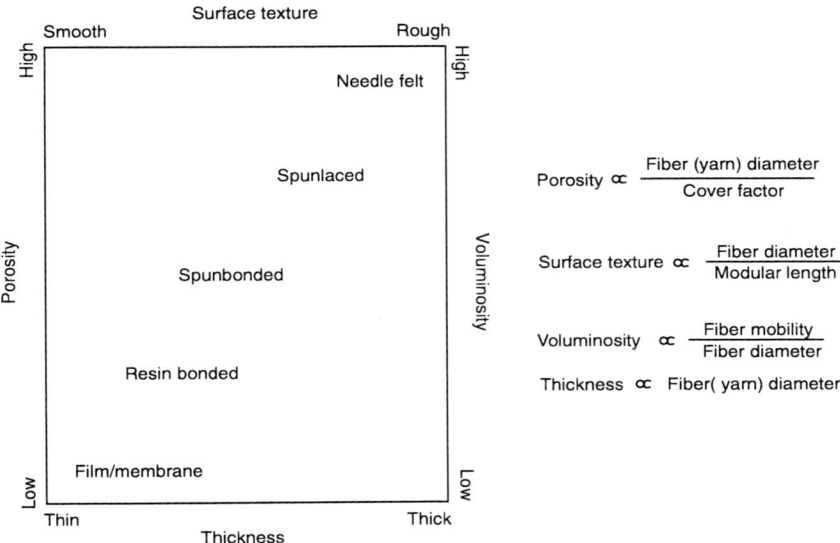

FIGURE B-7 Geometric properties of nonwoven fibers. Source: Ko and Song, 1996.

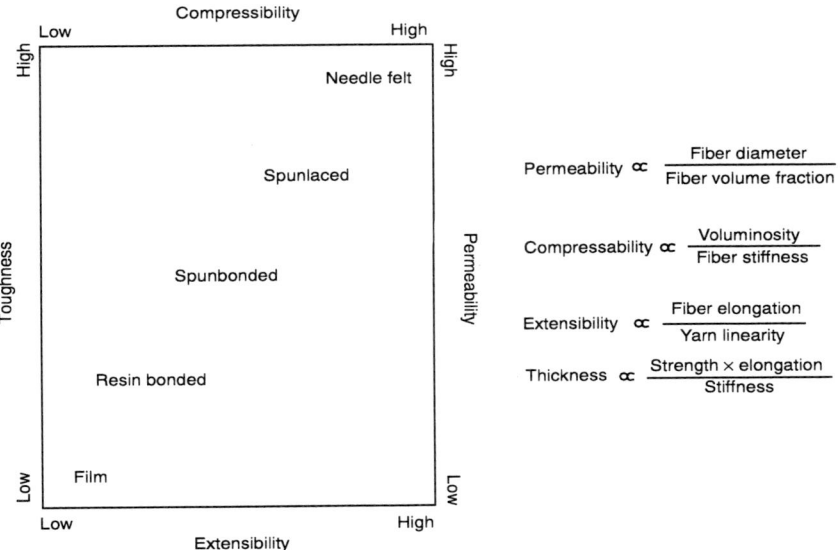

FIGURE B-8 Performance properties of nonwoven fibers. Source: Ko and Song, 1996.

For yarn in general, low permeability to air, vapor and light dictate;
1) High circularity coefficient for the component fibers;
2) Surface smoothness for the component fibers;
3) Low state of aggregation (packing factor) achieved, for example, by utilizing multiplanner crimp fibers and low twist.

For fabric in general, maximum translation of yarn properties for low permeability requires:
1) Low number of yarns per unit length and width of fabric;
2) Low cover factor factor-warp and filling;
3) High crimp level-warp and filling;
4) Maintenance of yarn circularity
5) Weave types containing the minimum number of continuous intersections.

High permeability requires essentially the converse of these characteristics.

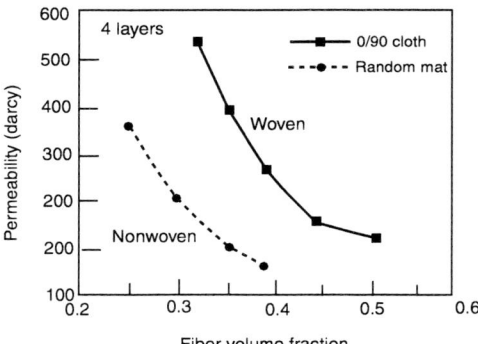

FIGURE B-9 Effects of fiber orientation on permeability. Source: Ko and Song, 1996.

have not been quantified or defined. New analytical methods will have to be developed for the new classes of fibrous materials and structures. Multifunctional materials will require special function polymeric fibers and hybrid yarns consisting of two or more polymers and their ultrafine filament derivatives. Yarns and fabrics consisting of the ultrafine fibers will require sophisticated processing and finishing techniques. The unique surface texture and multifunctional nature of these new textiles will require computer-aided design and manufacturing for reproducibility and flexible manufacturing for meeting mission-specific demands. The production economics will require high-speed, automated processes, including fiber spinning, fabric formation, printing (camouflage), and garment manufacturing. The capability of the U.S. defense industry to develop and field advanced CB protective textiles and garments will require the cooperative participation of research institutions as well as the fiber-textile-garment industry.

CONCLUSIONS

It is generally accepted that the impermeable system provides the most complete protection against CB agents, whereas the permeable system, which breathes and allows moisture vapor to escape, cannot protect against aerosol and liquid agents (Wilusz, 1998). Impermeable barriers, however, cause serious heat stress by trapping bodily moisture vapor inside the system. An incremental improvement can be achieved using a semipermeable barrier backed with a sorptive layer. This system allows

TABLE B-6 Trends In Chemical/Biological Protective Textiles

	Current	Future
Fiber material	Monofunctional	Multifunctional
Fiber geometry (diameter)	Micro >10µm	Nano <µm → nm
Fiber architecture (fabric)	Woven (yarn-to-fabric)	Nonwoven (hybrid) (fiber-to-fabric)
Garment manufacturing	Cut and sew labor intensive	Net shape, seamless automation, flexible manufacturing
Garment design	Skill based, sequential	Concurrent engineering, integrated
Characterization	Test and try	Continuous monitoring

Source: Ko, 1999.

the moisture vapor from the body to escape; however, air can still penetrate, and the system is both bulky and heavy.

An obvious solution would be ultrafine fibers (i.e., nanofibers or microfibers) for the membranes that could be selectively permeable. If one decreases the diameter to the nanoscale, the pore size of the membrane is reduced, and the available surface area is increased significantly. The strength of nanofiber fibers, however, is still far below that of conventional textile fibers. In addition, the technology of processing nanofibers in traditional textile machines is not well established. Neither the dynamic interaction between nanofibers and machine surfaces nor the problems that will be encountered in chemical and mechanical finishing of fabrics containing nanofibers (e.g., snagging, adhesion, melting, agglomeration) have been investigated.

The sewing process creates easy pathways for agent penetration. Therefore, the manipulation, transportation, and assembly of the protective garments must be carefully planned, whether the garment is made manually or automatically. A summary of the future directions in CB protective textile materials and technologies is presented in Table B-6.

A recent observation by Berkowitch (1996) describes the different approaches of the textile and apparel industries in the United States and Japan:

> The U.S. apparel industry's...strategy is driven mainly by cost, with yield, speed, and product uniformity at the top of its agenda and new

process development drastically reduced. Having gradually lost its equipment manufacturing segment, it relies on developments from foreign manufacturers for process modernization. The attention given to quality bears primarily on uniformity and processibility. Introduction of product variants is kept to a minimum and frequently prompted by pressure from imports in the lower half of the market. The mills have not been challenged by the specialty products covered in this report. These products are practically unavailable here because the currency exchange rate makes them exorbitantly expensive. The situation would likely change, though, were their prices to drop as a result of offshore manufacturing. Development of specialty products based on novel concepts has also been curtailed on the assumption that the U.S. consumer would not support the premium. The industry clearly continues to aim at a volume business and shows reluctance to diversify. Further evidence of this reluctance is found in the industry's phaseout of mid- and long-range research and in the focus of its limited technical resources on existing businesses. Both steps emphasize the overriding importance of short-term payoff.

Japanese and American strategies thus differ, and the contrast has grown over the years. Indeed, several developments presented in this report originated in the United States. But, as time went on, the industry here turned its attention elsewhere, while the Japanese latched onto the trends and improved on them. Time will tell which of the two will prevail in the barrier-free, fiercely cost- and quality-competitive world...

As these trends continue, the U.S. textile and garment industry will be dependent on foreign textile materials and machinery technology. If we wish to assess the readiness of the U.S. textile-garment industry to meet the CB protective textile and garment requirements, we must ask several questions. Do we have the necessary multifunctional fiber materials? Do we have the necessary specialty, ultrafine fiber, yarn, and fabric processing technologies? Do we have quick-response garment manufacturing technologies that can meet changing needs? Unfortunately, the answer to all of these questions is no.

Recognizing that U.S. industry is not prepared at the material or technological level to respond to the need for a selectively permeable uniform for the soldiers, the Department of Defense has taken the initiative by supporting R&D at universities and industry. Rapid advances in nanotechnology and biotechnology should stimulate the development of new material and processing concepts. New engineering design tools and manufacturing technologies will be necessary, however, for these innovative concepts to be translated into product realities.

References

Barrett, G. 1998. PM-ESS (Enhanced Soldier Systems) Managed Programs. Presentation by G. Barrett, Program Manager, Enhanced Soldier Systems, to principle investigators and members of the Advisory Panel on Strategies to Protect the Health of Deployed U.S. Forces, Task 2.3: Physical Protection and Decontamination. Solider and Biological Chemical Command, Natick, Massachusetts, November 16, 1999.

Berkowitch, J.E. 1996. Trends in Japanese Textile Technology. Washington, D.C.: U.S. Department of Commerce, Office of Technology Policy.

Brandler, P. 1998. State-of-the-Art of Functional Textiles for Soldiers' Related Systems, Functionally Tailored Textiles and Fabrics. Presented at the Second Annual Review Meeting, Army Research Laboratories, Aberdeen, Md., March 5–6, 1998.

DeWitt Smith, H., 1944. Textile Fibers: An Engineering Approach to their Properties and Utilization, Edgar Marburg Lecture. West Conshohocken, Pa.: American Society for Testing and Materials.

Fukuhara, M. 1993. Innovation in polymer fibers: from silk-like to new polyester. Textile Research Journal 63(7): 387–391.

Gander, T.J. 1997. Jane's NBC Protection Equipment, 10th ed. Surrey, U.K.: Jane's Information Group.

Gibson, P.W., H.L. Schreuder-Gibson, and D. Rivin. 1999. Electrospun fiber mats: transport properties. American Institute of Chemical Engineers Journal 45(1): 190–194.

Gibson, H. and D. Reneker. 1998. Nanofibers: New Fabric Architectures. Presentation to the U.S. Army Nanotechnology Conference, Boston, Massachusetts, July 7–9 1998.

Goswani, B., J.G. Martindale, and F.S. Scardino. 1971. Textile Yarns Technology: Structure and Applications. Springfield, Va.: National Technical Information Services.

Harris, M. 1954. Handbook of Textile Fibers. Washington, D.C.: Harris Research Laboratory, Inc.

Hidalgo, P. 1982. The Challenge of Chemical/Biological Warfare. Presentation by P. Hidalgo to the Outlook '82 IFAI 23rd Conference, New York, May 19, 1982.

Kaswell, E. 1965. Wellington Sears Handbook of Industrial Textiles. New York: Wellington Sears Company.

Ko, F.K. 1999. Textiles and Garments. Presentation by F.K. Ko, Drexel University, to principal investigators and members of the Advisory Panel on Strategies to Protect the Health of Deployed U.S. Forces, Task 2.3: Physical Protection and Decontamination. National Research Council, Washington, D.C., January 26, 1999.

Ko, F.K., and C.M. Pastore. 1985. Computer-Aided Design of Nonwoven Fabrics. Pp. 1–6 in Proceedings of the INDA Technical Symposium. New York: Association of the Nonwoven Fabrics Industry.

Ko, F.K., and J. Song. 1996. Chemical Protection Textiles. Presentation to the 3rd Textile Technology Workshop. Edgewood Research Development and Engineering Center and Drexel University, Philadelphia, Pennsylvania, December 4–5, 1996.

Ko, F.K., and A. Geshury. 1997. Liquid Chemical Agent Protection by Fabric Engineering. Final Report. Natick, Mass.: U.S. Army Natick Research Development & Engineering.

Ko, F.K., C.T. Laurencin, M.D. Borden, and D. Reneker. 1998. Dynamics of Cell Fiber Architecture Interaction. Pp. 11 in Proceedings of the Biomaterials Research Society Annual Meeting. San Diego, Calif.: Society of Biomaterials.

Mark, H., S. Atlas, and E. Ceria. 1967. Man-made Fibers: Science and Technology. New York: John Wiley and Sons.

McBriarty, J.P., and N.S. Henry. 1992. Performance of Protective Clothing. Vol. 4. ASTM STP 1133. West Conshohocken, Pa.: American Society for Testing and Materials.

Miller, B. 1986. Design Criteria for Effective Chemical Protective Clothing with Asymmetric Transport Properties. DAAK-60-83-C-0061. Natick, Mass.: U.S. Army Natick Research Development & Engineering.

Moncrieff, R.W. 1963. Man-made Fibers. New York: John Wiley and Sons.

Morris, J.V. 1977. Protective Clothing for Defense Purposes. Pp. 159–168 in Design of Textiles for Industrial Applications, P.W. Harrison, ed. Manchester, U.K.: Textile Institute.

Morton, W.E., and J.W.S. Hearle. 1975. Physical Properties of Textile Fibers. New York: John Wiley and Sons.

NRC (National Research Council). 1997. Technical Assessment of the Man-in-Simulant Test (MIST) Program. Board on Army Science and Technology, National Research Council. Board on Army Science and Technology. Washington, D.C.: National Academy Press.

Reneker, D.H., and I. Chun. 1996. Nanometer diameter fibers of polymer produced by electrospinning mats: transport properties. Journal of the American Institute of Chemical Engineers 45(1): 190–194.

Roth, R. 1982. Current Status of Research, Development, and Testing of Fabrics for Chemical/Biological Warfare. Presentation by R. Roth to the Outlook '82 IFAI 23rd Conference, New York, May 19, 1982.

U.S. Army. 1994. Army Science and Technology Master Plan, Fiscal Year 1995. Washington, D.C.: U.S. Army.

Wilusz, G. 1998. Science and Technology for Percutaneous Chemical and Biological Protection. Presentation by G. Wilusz, Chemical Technology Team, U.S. Army Soldier Systems Center, to principal investigators and members of the Advisory Panel on Strategies to Protect the Health of Deployed U.S. Forces, Task 2.3: Physical Protection and Decontamination. Soldier and Biological Chemical Command, Natick, Mass., November 16, 1998.

Appendix C

Evaluations of Barrier Creams[1]

Howard I. Maibach and Hongbo Zhai

IN VITRO DATA

In vitro studies test the effects of barrier creams on the skin, which mimics the reaction of in vivo skin. The in vitro method provides not only qualitative data (i.e., distinguishes between the creams) but also quantitative data (i.e., differences in absorption). Langford (1978) conducted in vitro studies to determine the behavior of a formulated fluorochemical-resin complex and a number of other solvents. He tested penetration through treated filter paper, repellency on treated pigskin, and penetration of radio-labeled sodium lauryl sulfate through treated hairless mouse skin. The fluorochemical-resin complex provided the best resistance against a range of solvents.

Reiner et al. (1982) studied the protective effect of model ointments on guinea pig skin in vitro. The permeation values of a toxic agent through unprotected and protected skin within 10 hours as a function of time were determined radiologically and enzymatically. Permeation of the toxic agent was markedly reduced by ointments with a polyethylene glycol base and ointments containing active substances.

Loden (1986) evaluated the effects of barrier creams on the absorption of (^{13}H)-water (^{14}C)-benzene and (^{14}C)-formaldehyde by excised human

---

[1]The following material was prepared for the use of the principal investigators of this study. The opinions and conclusions herein are the authors' and not necessarily those of the National Research Council.

skin. The control skins and treated skins were exposed to the test substance for 30 minutes, and the amount absorbed was determined. The model experimental "water barrier" cream reduced the absorption of water and benzene but not formaldehyde. Only one cream slightly reduced the absorption of benzene and formaldehyde; the others did not.

Fullerton and Menne (1995) tested the protective effect of ethylenediaminetetraacetate barrier gels against nickel contact allergy in *in vitro* and *in vivo* studies. In an *in vitro* study, about 30 mg of barrier gel was applied on the epidermal side of the skin and a nickel disc applied. After 24 hours, the disc was removed, the epidermis was separated from the dermis, and the nickel content in the epidermis and dermis was quantified by adsorption differential pulse voltammetry. The amount of nickel in the epidermal skin layer on treated skins was significantly less than the amount in untreated skins.

Zhai et al. (1999) used an *in vitro* diffusion system to measure the protective effect of quaternium-18 bentonite gels to prevent 1 percent concentration of [^{35}S] sodium lauryl sulfate penetration in human cadaver skin. The accumulated amount in receptor cell fluid was measured to evaluate the model gels over 24 hours. The test gels significantly decreased absorption when compared to the control samples of unprotected skin.

Treffel et al. (1994) measured the effectiveness on human skin of barrier creams against dyes (eosin, methylviolet, and oil red O) with varying n-octanol/water partition coefficients (0.19, 29.8 and 165, respectively). Barrier cream effects were assayed by measuring the dyes in the epidermis of protected skin samples after 30 minutes. They found no correlation between the galenic (pharmaceutic) parameters of the assayed products and the protection level, indicating that neither the water content nor the consistency of the formulations affected the level of protection. This physicochemical data could be used for tailoring barrier creams to meet the challenges of specific chemical agents.

IN VIVO DATA

Mahmoud and Lachapelle (1985) and Lachapelle et al. (1990) used a guinea pig model to evaluate the protective value of barrier creams and/or gels by laser Doppler flowmetry (blood flow) and histological assessment. The histopathological damage after 10 minutes of contact to toluene was mainly confined to the epidermis; the dermis was almost normal. Dermal blood flow changes were relatively high on the control site compared to the sites pretreated with gel. In addition, the blood concentrations of n-hexane in the control group and the gel-pretreated group were determined. It was possible to correlate results found by invasive (blood levels) and noninvasive techniques.

Frosch et al. (1993a, 1993b, 1993c), and Frosch and Kurte (1994) developed the repetitive irritation test in the guinea pig and in humans to evaluate barrier creams using a series bioengineering techniques. The pretreated and untreated test skin (guinea pig or human) was exposed daily to the irritants for two weeks. The resulting irritation was scored on a visual scale and assessed by biophysical (bioengineering) techniques. Some test creams suppressed irritation with all test parameters; some showed no effect, and even increased irritation.

Zhai and Maibach (1996) used an *in vivo* human model to measure the effectiveness of barrier creams against dye indicator solutions, methylene blue in water and oil red 0 in ethanol, representative of model hydrophilic and lipophilic compounds. Solutions of 5 percent methylene blue and 5 percent oil red O were applied to untreated and barrier-cream pretreated skin with the aid of aluminum occlusive chambers, for either a few minutes or four hours. At the end of the application time, the materials were removed and consecutive skin surface biopsies were taken. The amount of dye that had penetrated into each strip was determined by colorimetry. Two model creams were effective; one increased the cumulative amount of dye.

References

Frosch, P.J., A. Kurte, and B. Pilz, 1993a. Efficacy of skin barrier creams. 3. The repetitive irritation test (RIT) in humans. Contact Dermatitis 29: 113–118.

Frosch, P.J., A. Schultze-Dirks, M. Hoffmann, I. Axthelm, and A. Kurte. 1993b. Efficacy of skin barrier creams. 2. Ineffectiveness of a popular "skin protector" against various irritants in the repetitive irritation test in the guinea pig. Contact Dermatitis 29: 74–77.

Frosch, P.J., A. Kurte, and B. Pilz. 1993c. Biophysical Techniques for the Evaluation of Skin Protective Creams. Pp. 214–222 in Noninvasive Methods for the Quantification of Skin Functions. P.J. Frosch and A.M. Kligman, eds. Berlin: Springer-Verlag.

Frosch, P.J., and A. Kurte. 1994. Efficacy of skin barrier creams. 4. The repetitive irritation test (RIT) with a set of four standard irritants. Contact Dermatitis 31: 161–168.

Fullerton, A., and T. Menne. 1995. *In vitro* and *in vivo* evaluation of the effect of barrier gels in nickel contact allergy. Contact Dermatitis 32: 100–106.

Lachapelle J.M., H. Nouaigui, and L. Mavot. 1990. Experimental study of the effects of a new protective cream against skin irritation provoked by the organic solvents n-hexane, trichloethylene and toluene. Dermatosen Beruf Umwelt 38: 19–23.

Langford, N.P. 1978. Fluorochemical resin complexes for use in solvent repellent hand creams. American Industrial Hygiene Association Journal 39: 33–40.

Loden, M. 1986. The effect of four barrier creams on the absorption of water, benzene, and formaldehyde into excised human skin. Contact Dermatitis 14: 292–296.

Mahmoud, G., and J.M. Lachapelle. 1985. Evaluation of the protective value of an antisolvent gel by laser Doppler flowmetry and histology. Contact Dermatitis 13: 14–19.

Reiner, R., K. Rossmann, C.V. van Hooidonk, B.I. Cuelen, and J.Bock. 1982. Ointments for the protection against organophosphate poisoning. Arzneimittelforschung 32: 630–633.

Treffel, P., B. Gabard, and R. Juch. 1994. Evaluation of barrier creams: an in vitro technique on human skin. Acta Dermatologica Venereolica 74: 7–11.

Zhai, H., and H.I. Maibach. 1996. Effect of barrier creams: human skin *in vivo*. Contact Dermatitis 35: 92–96.

Zhai, H., D.J. Buddrus, A.A. Schultz, R.C. Wester, T. Hartway, S. Serianzana, and H.I. Maibach. 1999. In vitro percutaneous absorption of sodium lauryl sulfate in human skin decreased by quaternium-18 bentonite gels. *In Vitro* Molecular Toxicology 12: 11–15.

Appendix D

Evaluating Skin Decontamination Techniques[1]

Howard I. Maibach and Hongbo Zhai

Both *in vitro* and *in vivo* techniques have been developed to determine skin decontamination. A brief introduction to the models and a summary of the relative data from recent studies follows. The models described below have been developed with nonvesicant agents that are available for occupational and home use.

IN VIVO DECONTAMINATION MODEL

Wester et al. (1991) tested the extent and rate of decontamination on rhesus monkeys. A water-soluble chemical, glyphosate, was completely removed from rhesus monkey skin with three successive soap and water or water only washes. Approximately 90-percent of the glyphosate was removed in the first wash. There was no difference between washing with soap and water and washing with water only. Alachlor, a lipid-soluble chemical, was also removed by washing with soap and water and water only. In contrast to glyphosate, however, more alachlor was removed with soap and water than with water alone. Although the first alachlor washing removed most of the chemical, successive washings contributed to overall decontamination.

Methylene bisphenyl isocyanate, an industrial chemical, is a potent

---

[1]The following material was prepared for the use of the principal investigators of this study. The opinions and conclusions herein are the authors' and not necessarily those of the National Research Council.

contact sensitizer. Decontamination potential was determined *in vivo* in rhesus monkeys. A grid of 1-cm areas was drawn on the abdomen of the monkey (the same can be done with humans) and the same amount of chemical applied to all areas. At set times, individual grid areas were washed/decontaminated by water-only, 5-percent soap, 50-percent soap, polypropylene glycol, polypropylene glycol cleaner, and corn oil. After each washing procedure, skin tape stripping was used to quantify residual contamination. Water-only and soap-and-water washing were minimally effective. Polypropylene glycol, polypropylene glycol cleaner, and corn oil were more effective. The chemical that was not removed by the washing procedures was recovered in the tape stripping (Wester and Maibach, 1999a). Two factors affect *in vivo* skin decontamination: (1) the "rubbing effect" that removes loose surface stratum corneum from natural skin desquamation, and (2) the "solvent effect," which is related to chemical lipophilicity and may influence the washing effects (Wester et al., 1991).

van Hooidonk et al. (1983) evaluated a wide variety of common materials as skin decontaminants against chemical agents. Flour followed by wet tissue paper removed 93 percent of VX and 98 percent of mustard. This treatment also reduced the penetration of mustard (measured by radiolabel) and VX (measured by anti-acetylcholinesterase activity). *In vivo* tests confirmed a significant reduction in mortality with flour/ wet tissue paper after VX and soman exposures. The authors found that washing alone (with no flour pretreatment), either with water or soap and water, was highly effective against nerve agents, but resulted in much larger areas of skin damage for mustard. Therefore, the authors concluded that the best decontaminant for mustard, VX, and soman was decontamination with flour followed by an after-treatment with wet tissue.

IN VITRO DECONTAMINATION MODEL

In vitro skin mounted in diffusion cells can be decontaminated with solvents. The mounted skin is fragile, however, and cannot be rubbed as vigorously as *in vivo* skin. Another *in vitro* technique is mixing powdered human stratum corneum with radiolabeled formulations (Wester et al., 1987). For example, a water-only wash (and subsequent centrifugation) removed only 4.6 ± 1.3 percent of the "bound" alachlor. However, when the bound alachlor- powdered human stratum corneum was washed with 10-percent soap and water, 77.2 ± 5.7 percent was removed; with 50-percent soap and water, 90.0 ± 0.5 percent was removed. This model would predict that alachlor cannot be removed from the skin by washing with water alone but that soap will decontaminate the skin. The reason may be that the "lipid" constituents of soap offer a more favorable partitioning environment for the alachlor (Wester and Maibach, 1999b). These results were confirmed in *in vivo* studies. Large-scale *in vitro* decontamination screening can be done with the powdered human stratum corneum model.

In vitro studies conducted by decontaminating pig skin exposed to radiolabeled DFP (an organophosphorus compound, cholinesterase inhibitor) and radiolabeled n-butyl 2-choloroethylsulfide (a vesicant) compared the decontamination efficiency of a water shower (tap water), the M-258 kit, and a pad impregnated with a reactive resin mixture. Decontamination efficiencies were found to be similar for all three methods (Reifenrath, 1990). Shower decontamination with an aqueous surfactant solution did not increase the skin penetration of topically applied soman or thickened soman (Reifenrath et al., 1984).

References

Reinfenrath, W.G. 1990. *In vitro* determination of skin decontamination efficacy using a water shower. Toxicologist 10: 615.

Reifenrath, W.G., M.M. Mershon, F.B. Brinkley, G.A. Miura, C.A. Broomfield, and H.B. Cranford. 1984. Evaluation of diethyl malonate as a simulant for 1,2,2-trimethylpropyl methylphosphonofluoridate (soman) in shower decontamination of the skin. Journal of Pharmaceutical Science 73: 1388–1392.

van Hooidonk, C., B.I. Ceulen, J. Bock, and J. van Genderen. 1983. CW Agents and the Skin: Penetration and Decontamination. Pp. 153–160 in Proceedings of the International Symposium on Protection against Chemical Warfare Agents. Umea, Sweden: National Defence Research Institute.

Wester, R.C., M. Mobagen, and H.I. Maibach 1987. *In vivo* and *in vitro* absorption and binding to powered stratum corneum as methods to evaluate skin absorption of environmental chemical contaminants from ground and surface water. Journal of Toxicology and Environmental Health 21(3): 367–374.

Wester, R.C., J. Melendres, R. Sarason, J. McMaster, and H.I. Maibach. 1991. Glyphosate skin binding, absorption, residual tissue distribution, and skin decontamination. Fundamentals of Applied Toxicology 16: 725–732.

Wester, R.C., and H.I. Maibach. 1999a. *In Vivo* Methods for Percutaneous Absorption Measurements. Pp. 215–227 in Percutaneous Absorption, 3rd ed., R.L. Bronaugh and H.I. Maibach, eds. New York: Marcel Dekker, Inc.

Wester, R.C., and H.I. Maibach. 1999b. Dermal Decontamination and Percutaneous Absorption. Pp. 241–254 in Percutaneous Absorption, 3rd ed., R.L. Bronaugh and H.I. Maibach, eds. New York: Marcel Dekker, Inc.

Appendix E

Percutaneous Absorption[1]

Howard I. Maibach and Hongbo Zhai

IN VITRO PASSIVE DIFFUSION

Most *in vitro* techniques entail placing excised skin in a diffusion chamber, applying a chemical compound to its surface, and assaying the skin for the presence of the compound in the collection vessel on the other side. Excised human skin, animal skin, or artificial membranes can be used, and the skin may be intact or separated into epidermis and dermis (Wester and Maibach, 1993; Bronaugh, 1997; and Roberts et al., 1999). *In vitro* systems can be used to test the percutaneous absorption of chemicals that are too toxic to test in humans.

In vivo, the penetrating compound may not pass completely through the dermis but may be removed by metabolic mechanisms, such as through capillaries, and enter the blood stream causing systemic effects. With *in vitro* systems, skin metabolism can be studied in viable skin without interference from systemic metabolic processes. Absorption measurements can be obtained more easily from diffusion cells than from analyses of biological specimens from clinical studies. *In vitro* techniques are easy to use, and the results can be obtained rapidly. A disadvantage, however, is that the collection bath is saline, thus compatible with hydrophilic but not hydrophobic compounds.

---

[1]The following material was prepared for the use of the principal investigators of this study. The opinions and conclusions herein are the authors' and not necessarily those of the National Research Council.

COMPARTMENTAL MODELS

Compartmental models are alternatives to diffusion models of percutaneous absorption. Absorption of solute through the skin is generally assumed to follow first-order kinetics. Much of the data analyzed with compartmental models is characterized by "flip-flop" kinetics (i.e., the absorption half-time is much longer than the elimination half-time) (Roberts et al., 1999).

STRIPPING MODELS

Stripping models can be used to determine the concentration of chemicals in the stratum corneum at the end of a short application period (e.g., 30 minutes). First, the chemical is applied to skin of animals or humans. After 30 minutes, the stratum corneum is removed by successive applications of tape (Rougier et al., 1999; Surber et al., 1999). By linear extrapolation, stripping models can predict the percutaneous absorption of that chemical for longer periods. Rougier and coworkers (1986) established a linear relationship between the stratum corneum, reservoir content, and percutaneous absorption using the standard urinary excretion method (Feldmann and Maibach, 1967). The major advantages of the stripping method are: (1) absorption can be determined independent of urinary (and fecal) excretion; and (2) nonradiolabeled percutaneous absorption can be determined because the stripped skin samples contain enough chemical for modern chemical assay methods (Wester and Maibach, 1999a).

RADIOISOTOPIC TRACER METHODS

Radiolabeled compounds are widely used as tracers in both *in vitro* and *in vivo* studies. Many radiochemicals are commercially available; others may be synthesized to order. Radiochemicals are usually used to determine the amount of radioactivity in the "dermal"' compartment (receiver fluid) or in the skin compartment (epidermis, dermis).

Radiochemicals are also used to determine percutaneous absorption *in vivo* by the indirect method of measuring radioactivity in excreta (urine and feces) after topical application. Plasma radioactivity can be measured and the percutaneous absorption determined by the ratio of the areas under the plasma concentration to time curves following topical and intravenous administration (Wester and Maibach, 1999a). This method can detect low levels of chemical absorption.

ACCELERATOR MASS SPECTROMETER

Accelerator mass spectrometry (AMS) uses mass selection and energy gain to separate the isotope of carbon (and other elements) so that ions of the radioisotope can be counted. Tissue samples can be analyzed to quantify radioisotopes regardless of their decay times (Keating et al., 1999). AMS has distinct advantages over other methods of measuring percutaneous penetration. First, its analytic sensitivity is a thousand times greater than liquid scintillation counting (LSC). Therefore, flux determinations can be made using test chemicals at low enough concentrations to conduct human *in vivo* studies. AMS can also be used with other methods to quantify chemical absorption on tape strips after *in vivo* human dermal exposure (Keating et al., 1999).

Gilman et al. (1998) used AMS to detect ^{14}C-labeled urinary metabolites of atrazine (a triazine herbicide) and compared the analytical performance of AMS with LSC. Human subjects were given a dermal dose of ^{14}C-labeled atrazine over a 24-hour period. Urine samples from the subjects were collected over a seven-day period. The concentrations of ^{14}C in the samples determined by AMS and LSC ranged from 1.8 fmol/mL to 4.3 pmol/mL. The data from these two methods have a correlation coefficient of 0.998 for a linear plot of the entire sample set. AMS provides concentration (2.2 vs. 27 fmol/mL) and mass (5.5 vs. 54,000 amol) detection limits superior to those of LSC for these samples. The precision of the data provided by AMS for low-level samples is 1.7 percent; the day-to-day reproducibility of the AMS measurements is 3.9 percent.

REAL-TIME *IN VIVO* BIOAVAILABILITY

Wester and Maibach (1999a) used a real-time *in vivo* method to determine the bioavailability of organic solvents following dermal exposure. Breath analysis was used to obtain real-time measurements of volatile organic compounds in expired air following exposure. Human volunteers and animals breathed fresh air via a breath inlet system for continuous real-time analysis of undiluted exhaled air. The air supply system was self-contained and separated from the exposure solvent-laden environment. The system used an ion-trap mass spectrometer equipped with an atmospheric sampling glow discharge ionization source. The ion-trap mass spectrometer system was used to measure individual chemical components in the breath stream in the single-digit parts per billion detectable range for each of the compounds proposed for study, while maintaining linearity of response over a wide dynamic range.

OCCLUSION

Occlusion is covering the applied dose, either intentionally (e.g., bandaging) or unintentionally (e.g., putting on clothing) after applying a topical agent. A vehicle such as an ointment can also have occlusive properties. Occlusion results in a combination of many physical factors that affect the skin and the applied compound by enhancing hydration and sometimes increasing skin temperature. Occlusion also prevents the accidental wiping or evaporation of the applied compound, in essence ensuring a higher applied dose. Occlusion increases flux and is synergistic with skin damage (Wester and Maibach, 1983). Occlusion is a practical clinical method of enhancing percutaneous absorption, which suggests that its use in chemical defense should be studied further.

The relationship between occlusion and rate of penetration depends on the solubility of the penetrant. Furthermore, the extent of penetration may depend on the method of occlusion (Bucks and Maibach, 1999).

REGIONAL VARIATION

Feldmann and Maibach (1967) systematically investigated regional variations in percutaneous absorption and found that the absorption of hydrocortisone differed at different anatomical sites. The scrotum was the highest absorbing skin site and the sole of the foot the lowest. Other studies have also focused on the influence of anatomical site on the absorption of various drugs and chemicals in humans and in animals (Wester and Maibach, 1999b). For example, scopolamine transdermal systems are placed in the postauricular area because an effective amount of the drug is absorbed at this site.

Mathematical models are used to estimate human health hazards of environmental contaminants even though data may be available for only one anatomic site. With toxicants on the exposed areas of the skin (head, face, and neck), flux will be greater than on glabrous skin. Estimates of skin absorption rates are integral to estimates of potential hazards (Wester and Maibach, 1999b).

ANIMAL VERSUS HUMAN STUDIES

Human skin is unique, and the structural differences in various animal species may or may not affect the penetrability of a specific compound. Numerous *in vivo* and *in vitro* studies have been conducted comparing percutaneous absorption in animal and human skin. In general, the skin of monkeys (rhesus and squirrel) and weanling pig most resembles human skin. The skin of rats and rabbits is more permeable than human skin. Animals can be used to generate kinetic data; but no one animal skin can simulate the percutaneous penetration in humans for all compounds. Therefore, the best estimates of human percutaneous absorption are based on *in vivo* experiments on humans (Zhai and Maibach, 1996).

IN VITRO VERSUS *IN VIVO* STUDIES

Methods of *in vitro* percutaneous absorption are widely used to measure the absorption of topically applied compounds. A major advantage of *in vitro* systems is that they can be used to test compounds that are too toxic to test in humans. Metabolism can be measured if viable skin is obtained and the viability is maintained in the diffusion cells (Wester et al., 1998). Skin metabolism can be studied in viable skin without interference from systemic metabolic processes (Bronaugh et al., 1999). Finally, absorption measurements can be made more easily from diffusion cells than from analyses of biological specimens from clinical studies.

In vitro methods are simple, rapid, and safe and are recommended as a first step in defining percutaneous absorption. The major disadvantages of *in vitro* tests are: (1) excised (and usually stored) skin may not retain full enzymatic activity; (2) drug metabolism probably does not affect the amount of compound entering the stratum corneum, but it may affect the metabolic profile emerging from the skin; (3) the collection bath is saline, which is compatible with hydrophilic compounds but not with hydrophobic compounds; and (4) *in vivo*, the penetrating compound does not pass completely through the dermis but is removed by dermal capillaries (Wester and Maibach, 1983). Because of notable differences between *in vivo* and *in vitro* skin, the *in vitro* method alone is not always a reliable or accurate predictor of *in vivo* percutaneous absorption.

References

Bronaugh, R. L. 1997. Methods for *In Vitro* Percutaneous Absorption. Pp. 7–14 in Dermatotoxicology Methods: The Laboratory Worker's *Vade Mecum*. Washington, D.C.: Taylor and Francis.

Bronaugh, R., H. Hood, M. Kraeling, and J. Yourick. 1999. Determination of Percutaneous Absorption by *In Vitro* Techniques. Pp. 229–233 in Percutaneous Absorption, 3rd ed., R.L. Bronaugh and H.I. Maibach, eds. New York: Marcel Dekker, Inc.

Bucks, D., and H.I. Maibach. 1999. Occlusion Does Not Uniformly Enhance Penetration *In Vivo*. Pp. 81–105 in Percutaneous Absorption, 3rd ed., R.L. Bronaugh and H.I. Maibach, eds. New York: Marcel Dekker, Inc.

Feldmann, R.J., and H.I. Maibach. 1967. Regional variation in percutaneous penetration of ^{14}C cortisol in man. Journal of Investigative Dermatology 48(2): 181–183.

Gilman, S.D., S.J. Gee, B.D. Hammock, J.S. Vogel, K. Haack, B.A. Buchholz, S.P. Freeman, R.C. Wester, X. Hui, and H.I. Maibach. 1998. Analytical performance of accelerator mass spectrometry and liquid scintillation counting for detection of ^{14}C-labeled atrazine metabolites in human urine. Analytical Chemistry 70(16): 3463–3469.

Keating, G.A., K.T. Bogen, and J.S. Vogel. 1999. Measurement of short-term dermal uptake *in vitro* using accelerator mass spectrometry. Pp. 475–486 in Percutaneous Absorption, 3rd ed., R.L. Bronaugh and H.I. Maibach, eds. New York: Marcel Dekker, Inc.

Roberts, M.S., Y.G. Anissimov, and R.A. Gonsalvez. 1999. Mathematical models in percutaneous absorption. Pp. 3–55 in Percutaneous Absorption, 3rd ed., R.L. Bronaugh and H.I. Maibach, eds. New York: Marcel Dekker, Inc.

Rougier, A., D. Dupuis, C. Lotte, R.C. Wester, and H.I. Maibach. 1986. Regional variation in percutaneous absorption in man: measurement by the stripping method. Archives of Dermatology Research 278: 465–469.

Rougier, A., D. Dupuis, C. Lotte, and H.I. Maibach. 1999. Stripping method for measuring percutaneous absorption *in vivo*. Pp. 375–394 in Percutaneous Absorption, 3rd ed., R.L. Bronaugh and H.I. Maibach, eds. New York: Marcel Dekker, Inc.

Surber, C., F.P. Schwarb, and E.W. Smith. 1999. Tape-stripping technique. Pp. 395–409 in Percutaneous Absorption, 3rd ed., R.L. Bronaugh and H.I. Maibach, eds. New York: Marcel Dekker, Inc.

Wester, R.C., and H.I. Maibach. 1983. Cutaneous pharmacokinetics: ten steps to percutaneous absorption. Drug Metabolism Review 14: 169–205.

Wester, R.C., and H.I. Maibach. 1993. Topical Drug Delivery: Percutaneous Absorption. Pp. 3–15 in Topical Drug Bioavailability, Bioequivalence, and Penetration, V.P. Shah, and H.I. Maibach, eds. New York: Plenum Press.

Wester, R.C., J. Christoffel, T. Hartway, N. Poblete, H.I. Maibach, and J. Forsell. 1998. Human cadaver skin viability for *in vitro* percutaneous absorption: storage and detrimental effects of heat-separation and freezing. Pharmacology Research 15(1): 82–84.

Wester, R.C., and H.I. Maibach. 1999a. *In Vivo* Methods for Percutaneous Absorption Measurements. Pp. 215–227 in Percutaneous Absorption, 3rd ed., R.L. Bronaugh and H.I. Maibach, eds. New York: Marcel Dekker, Inc.

Wester, R.C., and H.I. Maibach. 1999b. Regional Variation in Percutaneous Absorption. Pp. 107–116 in Percutaneous Absorption, 3rd ed., R.L. Bronaugh and H.I. Maibach, eds. New York: Marcel Dekker, Inc.

Zhai, H., and H.I. Maibach. 1996. Pp. 193–205 in Prevention of Contact Dermatitis, Current Problems in Dermatology, P. Elsner, J.M Lachapelle, J. E. Wahlberg, and H.I. Maibach, eds. New York: Karger.

Appendix F

Contributors to This Study

Gloria Akins
CBIAC

MAJ Michael Avery
U.S. Army Chemical School

James Baker
SBCCOM
Edgewood Chemical Biological Center

Gloria Barrett
SBCCOM
Soldier Systems Center

LTC Roger Baxter
USAMRICD

Carolyn Bensel
SBCCOM
Soldier Systems Center

John Birkner
TWP4, DIA

Andy Blankenbiller
JSMG

MAJ Graeme Boyett
Office of the Special Assistant for Gulf War Illnesses

Robert Boyle
Boyle Productions

Kelley Brix
Office of the Special Assistant for Gulf War Illnesses

Linda Brown
National Ground Intelligence Center

COL Mike Brown
Joint Staff

Rinaldo Bucci
SBCCOM
Edgewood Chemical Biological Center

James Byrnes
SBCCOM
Edgewood Chemical Biological Center

Bruce Cadarette
USARIEM

Thomas Cardella
Office of the Special Assistant for Gulf War Illnesses

David Caretti
SBCCOM
Edgewood Chemical Biological Center

LTC Katie Carr
Commodity Area Manager

Brian Corner
SBCCOM
Soldier Systems Center

Wayne Davis
SBCCOM
Edgewood Chemical Biological Center

Joseph DeFrank
SBCCOM
Edgewood Chemical Biological Center

Al Dickson
STI

Mildred Donlon
DARPA

Ann Dufresne
Nonproliferation Center, CIA

Bill Eck
TWP5, DIA

David English
ILC Dover

CAPT Daniel Farmer
U.S. Army Chemical School

John Ferriter
SBCCOM
Edgewood Chemical Biological Center

Gyleen Fitzgerald
SBCCOM
Edgewood Chemical Biological Center

Cheri Foust
Oak Ridge National Laboratory

Nicole Funk
Booz-Allen & Hamilton, Inc.

COL C.R. Galles
SBCCOM
Edgewood Chemical Biological Center

Henry Gardner
USACEHR
Ft. Detrick

Karl Gerhart
SBCCOM
Edgewood Chemical Biological Center

Roger L. Gibbs
Naval Surface Warfare Center
Dahlgren Division

Margaret Graf
Office of the Special Assistant for
Gulf War Illnesses

Will Hartzell
Individual Protection,
Commodity Area Manager

Veronique Hauschild
USACHPPM

Jack Heller
USACHPPM

Richmond Henriques
Office of the Special Assistant for
Gulf War Illnesses

Matthew Herz
SBCCOM
Soldier Systems Center

William Hinds
University of California, Los
Angeles

Amoretta Hoeber
AMH Consulting

Tamra Ince
SBCCOM
Edgewood Chemical Biological
Center

Richard F. Johnson
USARIEM

CAPT Bill Karatzas
U.S. Army Chemical School

CAPT Michael Kilpatrick
Office of the Special Assistant for
Gulf War Illnesses

MAJ Larry Kimm
J-4 Logistics Directorate
Medical Readiness
Division

James King
CBIAC

MAJ Joe Kiple
Decontamination, Commodity
Area Manager

Charles Kirkwood
U.S. Army Chemical
School

CDR Paul Knechtges
USACEHR
Ft. Detrick

Wade Kuhlmann
SBCCOM
Edgewood Chemical Biological
Center

Brad Laprise
SBCCOM
Soldier Systems Center

MAJ Erich Lehnert
USAMRICD

COL Little
USA MRICD

Brian MacIver
SBCCOM
Edgewood Chemical Biological
Center

Dale Malabarba
SBCCOM
Soldier Systems Center

APPENDIX F

MAJ Mallamaci
U.S. Army Chemical School

Elizabeth McCoy
SBCCOM
Soldier Systems Center

James McKivrigan
Director, Executive Office
for the JSMG

Sirvart Mellian
Navy Clothing and Textile
Research Facility

Ken Miller
U.S. Army Chemical School

Miles Miller
SBCCOM
Edgewood Chemical Biological
Center

Dee Dodson Morris
Office of the Special Assistant for
Gulf War Illnesses

Robert Morrison
SBCCOM
Edgewood Chemical Biological
Center

Adolfo Negron
SBCCOM
Edgewood Chemical Biological
Center

Kelly Niernberger
Office of the Special Assistant for
Gulf War Illnesses

COL Pat Nilo
HQDA, ODCSOPS

COL Francis O'Donnell
Office of the Special Assistant for
Gulf War Illnesses

John O'Keefe
SBCCOM
Soldier Systems Center

MAJ Jonathan Payne
U.S. Army Chemical School

CAPT Mary Payton
U.S. Army Chemical
School

Thomas Pease
Gentex

Brad Perkins
U.S. Army Chemical School

Kirkman Phelps
Contamination Avoidance,
Commodity Area Manager

Amy Polcyn
SBCCOM
Soldier Systems Center

Michael Pompeii
Collective Protection,
Commodity Area Manager

SFC Jason Potter
Office of the Special Assistant for
Gulf War Illnesses

John Pullo
Gentex

Ellen Raber
Lawrence Livermore National
Laboratory

Ludwig Rebenfeld
Textile Research Institute

Gary Resnick
SBCCOM
Edgewood Chemical Biological Center

John Resta
CHPPM

Roy Reuter
Life Systems

Brad Roberts
Institute for Defense Analyses

COL James Romano
USAMRICD

Bob Rose
Hemispheric Center for Environmental Technology

James Savage
SBCCOM
Edgewood Chemical Biological Center

H. Schreuder–Gibson
SBCCOM
Soldier Systems Center

Doug Schultz
Institute for Defense Analyses

John Scully
JSIG

Kris Senecal
SBCCOM
Soldier Systems Center

Mark Shifflett
SBCCOM
Edgewood Chemical Biological Center

Eddie Shuff
National Ground Intelligence Center

Jack Siegel
SBCCOM
Soldier Systems Center

Jane Simpson
SBCCOM
Soldier Systems Center

Page Stoutland
DOE
Office of Nonproliferation and National Security

Maher Tadros
Sandia National Laboratory

R. Steven Tharratt
University of California
Davis Medical Center

Greg Thomas
Sandia National Laboratory

COL Thompson
U.S. Army Chemical School

Richard Traeger
Sandia National Laboratory

Russ Travers
DIA

COL Daniel Uyesugi
U.S. Army Chemical School

John Wallace
OIC
Naval Research Laboratory Detachment

John Weimaster
SBCCOM
Edgewood Chemical Biological Center

Matthew Whipple
SBCCOM
Soldier Systems Center

William White
SBCCOM
Edgewood Chemical Biological Center

COL Stan Wiener
DIA Science and Technology Advisory Board

Roy Williams
U.S. Army Chemical School

John Wilson
U.S. Army Chemical School

Eugene Wilusz
SBCCOM
Soldier Systems Center

Lynn Yang
Institute for Defense Analyses

Nick Yura
SBCCOM
Edgewood Chemical Biological Center

Kaveh Zamani
DDR&E

Jim H. Zarzycki
SBCCOM
Edgewood Chemical Biological Center

Alan Zelicoff
Sandia National Laboratory

Hongbo Zhai
University of California, San Francisco

Appendix G

Biographical Sketches of Principal Investigators and Members of the Advisory Panel

PRINCIPAL INVESTIGATORS

DR. MICHAEL KLEINMAN is Associate Director of the Air Pollution Effects Laboratory and Adjunct Professor at the Department in Community and Environmental Medicine at the School of Medicine, University of California, Irvine. Dr. Kleinman's research program examines the mechanisms by which inhaled toxic chemicals, alone and in mixtures, interfere with the cardiopulmonary system and with respiratory system defenses, using both laboratory animals and human subjects. Dr. Kleinman is chair of the State of California Environmental Protection Agency Air Quality Advisory Committee, a former member of the Toxicology Committee of the American Industrial Hygiene Association, and a member of the U.S. EPA's Science Advisory Board Health and Economic Effects Subcommittee. Dr. Kleinman is also a member of the Human Subjects Research Committee and the Biosafety Committee at the University of California-Irvine.

DR. MICHAEL WARTELL is Chancellor of the Indiana University-Purdue University Fort Wayne with a Ph.D. in Physical Chemistry from Yale University. He was involved in the Army Science Board in the 1980's where issues of chemical and biological defenses were part of Ad Hoc and Summer Study Groups in which he participated. In 1997, he rejoined the Army Science Board and is an ex-officio member of the Defense Science Board. He also serves as chair of the Defense Intelligence Agency Science and Technology Advisory Board. His positions on these boards are unpaid and afford a broad view of current activities with regard to protection against chemical and biological warfare. Dr. Wartell is interested in defense issues related to chemical and biological warfare and DoD policies and doctrine.

ADVISORY PANEL

WYETT H. COLCLASURE II is a retired Colonel with the U.S. Army who received his M.S. in Chemistry from the University of Illinois. He is currently the Chairman of the Environmental Technologies Group, Inc. Col. (ret.) Colclasure held many important positions within the Army including Project Manager for NBC Defense Systems of the Chemical and Biological Defense Command, Aberdeen Proving Ground; Director of Materiel Test, Dugway Proving Ground, and; Chief of the Chemical Operations Division, HQ Army Materiel Command. He has conducted the analyses of environmental studies, led a field and lab testing organization, prepared Department of Defense reports for Congress and directed the writing of concepts used to guide development of new chemical defense doctrine and equipment.

STEPHEN R. HILL received his Ph.D. in Public Policy and International Relations from the University of Maryland. Dr. Hill is the President of Global Analytics, Inc. which was awarded a multi-year sole source contract in support of the Data Fusion Facility for systems integration. His prior work experience includes TASC, Inc. were he was the principle investigator in the USAF preparedness for nuclear, biological and chemical warfare attacks, counter-proliferation, application of non-linear sciences to geopolitical issues, and strategic stability for the Strategic Defense Initiative Organization/Ballistic Missile Defense Organization. He has co-authored a Report to Congress describing the deployment plan for the ballistic missile defense and authored a book entitled *Fostering High Technology Industries: Firm Behavior, Industry Structure and National Policy*.

SIDNEY A. KATZ graduated with a Ph.D. in analytical chemistry from the University of Pennsylvania. Dr. Katz is currently a Professor in the Department of Chemistry, Rutgers University. His areas of research include the role and fate of trace elements in environmental and biological systems and the identification of toxic substances in the domestic and occupational environments. Awards that he has received include a NATO Senior Fellowship in Science, Army Research Associateships, USIS Lectureships and a Fulbright Lectureship. Dr. Katz has published extensively including a dozen technical reports prepared for agencies such as the U.S. Army Chemical and Biological Defense Agency, the New Jersey State Department of Environmental Protection and the International Agency Energy Agency.

FRANK KO received a Ph.D. in Polymer Science and Textile Engineering from the Georgia Institute of Technology and is currently a professor of Materials Engineering at Drexel University. In addition, he is the Director of the Fibrous Materials Research Center and on the Core Faculty of the Biomedical Institute. His research interests include the technology and modeling of textile structural composites, fiber viscoelasticity, the engineering design of medical and industrial textiles, the engineering design and processing of 3-D scaffolds for tissue engineering, and the engineering properties of high performance fibers. Dr. Ko serves on the editorial boards of the *Journal of Composites Technology and Research, Journal of Nonwoven Research, Composites,* and *Applied Sciences and Manufacturing.* He has also served as a committee member for the Assessment of the U.S. Army Natick Research, Development and Engineering Center and a proposal reviewer for the Army Research Office and the National Science Foundation.

HOWARD MAIBACH received his M.D. from Tulane University and an honorary Ph.D. from the University of Paris. Dr. Maibach currently serves as a professor in the Department of Dermatology at the University of California School of Medicine. His areas of research include dermatotoxicology, dermatopharmacology and environmental dermatoses. He has previously served on the Committee on Toxicology, Committee on Protection against Mycotoxins, Panel on Irritant Chemicals, and the Coordinating Committee to the Subcommittee on Possible Long-term Effects of Short Term Exposures to Chemical Agents. Dr. Maibach has authored or co-authored over 1,400 publications and 50 books in his area of expertise.

NAJMEDIM MESHKATI graduated with a Ph.D. in industrial and systems engineering from the University of Southern California (USC). Dr. Meshkati is an associate professor of civil/environmental engineering and associate professor of industrial and systems engineering at USC. He is the former associate director of the Institute of Safety and Systems Management (ISSM) where he was responsible for Professional Programs which included the 46-year old USC aviation safety, transportation safety management and occupational safety and health continuing education programs. Dr. Meshkati is an elected fellow of the Human Factors and Ergonomics Society and was a recipient of the Presidential Young Investigator Award for the National Science Foundation. His technical reports and articles on safety, health and environment; risk management, ergonomics and safety of petrochemical plants and nuclear power stations; and aviation safety have been published, disseminated and cited by many United Nations specialized agencies.